T0209732

87DAYS

STACY CLORAN

BALBOA.
PRESS

A DIVISION OF HAY HOUSE

Balboa Press books may be ordered through booksellers or by contacting:

Balboa Press
A Division of Hay House
1663 Liberty Drive
Bloomington, IN 47403
www.balboapress.com
1 (877) 407-4847

ISBN: 978-1-9822-2055-6 (sc)
ISBN: 978-1-9822-2064-8 (e)

Print information available on the last page.

Balboa Press rev. date: 01/24/2019

Dedication

This book is dedicated to my son, whose courage, strength and absolute unwillingness to throw in the towel continues to inspire me to this day. He beat the odds again and again no matter the challenge or the difficulty. He can literally light up a room with his contagious belly laugh and he has had the most phenomenal and unprecedented impact on my life. I love you so much little man.

Intro

People have been telling me for years that I should write a book, mostly my mom, but friends, colleagues and strangers too. I always brushed off the idea. I'm not a famous celebrity and I really didn't think my life was that interesting. I felt like those who thought it was needed to get out more! Then I was put in solitary confinement (aka bed rest) where I had A LOT of time to think, and I came to the conclusion that I guess I have had some pretty unique experiences, both good and bad and some just bizarre. If nothing else, I hope some of the stories bring a smile to your face and help you get through whatever you're going through. All the stories are true, and they happened to me. Granted, some of them happened during my young, crazy days so the details might be a little fuzzy (from being tired from studying so hard.... really mom and dad) but the basics are still there. I have of course changed the names of the other parties involved to protect their privacy.

I set up the book in two parts. The first part is about my dreadful experience during my sentence of hospitalized bed rest and the second part is full of short stories to entertain you (especially if you're on bed rest too, I love a captive audience!) Most of the stories are animal related because my entire life has revolved around them. I started working in a vet clinic at 13 years old and then became a Registered Veterinary Technician at 21 and never looked back. There are other stories too, so don't despair if you're not all that fond of animal hair on your jeans.

87 DAYS

Part 1

CHAPTER 1

I woke up just before dawn, stretched and quickly realized that my lower half was soaked. I leapt out of bed, looked at the drenched sheets and ran to the bathroom. Waking up in this state would be concerning for anyone but I was pregnant and nowhere near due yet. Twenty- three weeks and two days along, to be exact. I let out a yell and we busted ass to get dressed and get to the teeny-weenie hospital 20 minutes away.

Upon arrival, we were the only ones there and the nurse was visibly nervous. She had paged the on-call Dr and he was on his way. In the meantime, I donned my butt-flap gown and anxiously waited. He arrived wearing flip flops and cargo shorts - not instilling a lot of confidence in me. He went about the pelvic exam, said he saw nothing wrong and patronizingly patted my knee and said, "Don't worry dear, lots of pregnant women lose bladder control." My partner at the time stifled a chuckle and shrunk back into the corner because he knew this guy was about to get his ass chewed out. I did not disappoint. I know my body. I certainly know the difference between urine and amniotic fluid. I knew he was incompetent. And I knew that my intuition was ringing every possible warning bell to get my attention.

As soon as I discovered I was pregnant I had been referred to a high-risk OB/GYN team a few hours away in a very large city. You see, I was no spring chicken at the time and I was also dealing with lupus. Because of our very rural location, I had a nurse practitioner as my primary care giver and made regular trips to the specialists. After redressing, we drove straight to those specialists, with me cursing and leaking the whole way. The doctors saw me right away and diagnosed me with PPROM (premature rupture of membrane). It was beyond serious. As the dirty 7 letter word (bedrest) was thrown around I was one unhappy camper. I tried ignoring it, pretending there had been some mistake, pretending they were talking about someone else, getting angry, getting scared out of my mind. Alas, my denial was for naught, because there was no way around it. The doctors said if I could find a place to stay close to the hospital for the next few days and agreed to come in every day for a check up, they wouldn't admit me until I reached 24 weeks. The reason was depressing. They said they couldn't do much to help the baby if they're born younger than that. Lucky for me, my friend's house was about 7 minutes away and she and her husband generously offered for me to stay there. Thank God, Buddha, Allah, the Universe for Annabel and Sebastian. Not only for the accommodations, but for providing me a safe place to deal with the raging emotions, fear and panic. Between the 2 of them, they saved me from insanity daily. Everything from listening endlessly with compassion to playing the hang drum for me to try to help relax me. Dudes, seriously, THANK YOU.

It was a very scary week of rushing in and out of emerge. By the last day of "freedom", I had started hemorrhaging and I was out of options. It's funny how everything is relative and can be put into perspective with only a few words....

"You are being admitted to the hospital for strictly monitored bedrest for the duration of your pregnancy."

I heard, "Blah, blah, blah MAXIMUM SECURITY LOCKDOWN. Hahahaha (evil laugh)

I panicked. I was nauseous, dizzy, claustrophobic, I broke into a cold sweat and my mind raced through all the thousands of reasons why I simply could not be locked up for 4 1/2 months. I actually started looking around and planning how I could escape without anyone tackling me. Don't get me wrong, my unborn baby was my top priority, but I've always been a 100 mile/hr 24/7 person who despises laziness and rarely sits down and relaxes. I've always figured that if I'm awake, I should be doing something productive. Of course, growing a healthy baby is about as productive as you can be but during those moments I was not thinking rationally.

That day, sitting in emerge, waiting for the nurses to do the paperwork was awful. I felt like I was waiting for the hangman to tighten my noose. My body and mind had gone into a sort of mild shock state. I was zoned right out but could still follow their instructions in a detached way (sign here, etc.).

They pulled blood and hooked me up to an IV line and then brought me to my room. In hindsight, I was very lucky because the hospital had just opened a brand-new wing for ladies in my position. Apparently, the previous accommodations had been pretty poor. They gave me a room with 3 big windows.... that didn't open to allow air in, or me out. It's almost cruel and unusual punishment to provide a view of outside/normal life and freedom when it is unattainable. Maybe instead of putting prisons in desolate, isolated areas, they should put them in the middle of everything, so the bad guys have a constant reminder of what they're missing. I believe it would give them a whole lot more incentive to behave and get back to a real life.

The environment was so sterile (yes, I'm aware that's a good thing in a hospital), depressing and scary. It was a huge departure from my home in the country, on 50 acres of bush, with my horses, my dogs, nature and wildlife. There are no words in the English language to adequately express my despair that day. I had never experienced such fear and hopelessness or felt so impotent in my life.

During the next 87 days, I experienced many, many things that I wouldn't wish on my worst enemy, but I won't focus too much on them now (unless I can find some humor in them) because I want to help you through your bed rest, not scare or upset you.

The Meeting

My pregnancy journey had been a bumpy one to say the least up to the point of being admitted for hospitalized bed rest.

At one of my very early ultrasounds, I remember laying on the table with the globs of freezing cold goo sliding down my sides, watching the technicians face with CIA intensity. She tried her best to keep a non-reactive face, but I could tell something was wrong. I tried to ask a few times what was going on, but she would just smile and give a generic answer like "the baby isn't co-operating" or "it's tricky to get this view". She did finally say that this ultrasound does take longer than the previous ones because she had to take some measurements, so I relaxed a little but not much. She finished and went to get her superior - shit. The boss repeated some of the views and told me that the results would be sent to my specialist soon but that she of course could tell me nothing. I left in tears, feeling very alone, scared and helpless.

Soon after I was called back to have an appointment with my doctor. It was the WORST day ever. She came in, put her hand on my knee and proceeded to tell me that there were many problems with my baby. I don't remember all the medical terminology, but there were problems with his heart, they couldn't find his bladder, he had a large bubble on his brain and I had a low amount of amniotic fluid (this is before my water broke). Each one alone was very serious but all 4 together was a veritable death sentence. I shattered. With sincere compassion, she instructed my son's father and I to go home and "come to terms with what she told us and to make arrangements". We were to come back the following week to see her again. I cannot put into words what was going on in my head, my heart and my world. I felt like such a failure. What was wrong with me? What did I do wrong? We had a tearful weekend and even picked out a memorial spot on our property. There were very few words spoken, except for confirming with each other that we had both heard all the same facts and prognosis. I even had a few beers that weekend out of desperation to not feel the horrendous feelings raging in me. I had had a completely dry pregnancy up until then and continued to after that weekend. I also continued to give myself guilt over those few beers to this very day but at that dark time I figured that all was lost and was clawing at anything to provide some comfort.

We headed back to the hospital a few days later and were met with an unwelcome surprise. The young nurse who was the first to see us in the room, was perky and asked how I was doing. I looked at her stunned and refreshed her memory on the situation. She was embarrassed and quickly left the room. Then we were having a meeting with 5 specialists at the top of their field - a geneticist, a surgeon, a pediatrician, a NICU doctor and a doctor specializing in children with special needs. It was a tiny office and very crowded. All eyes were on me and they all gave their opinions - which were all the same - abortion because they all felt my baby had no chance. I swallowed my raging river of emotion and fired back many, many questions, which were met by surprise. I don't think any of them were used to being questioned but if I had learned anything from my years of my own medical issues and misdiagnoses it is to stand up for yourself and be your own health advocate. I vehemently refused their advice and for the first time in my life I listened to my body. It was telling me without a shadow of a doubt to ignore them. Like when you get the feeling that someone is watching you or is bad news - you don't question it you get the hell out of Dodge. That's how concrete this feeling was, and it encompassed my whole body, starting deep in my belly. Against all the so-called facts, I was not giving up on this little guy. I left there with a new-found fire lit under me. Maybe it was the old stubborn, firecracker teenage me coming back or maybe it was the new protective mama bear that was rapidly developing - I didn't know but I liked it and I grabbed onto it with both hands.

Soon after this excruciating ordeal, my water broke extremely early and I was admitted. However, I NEVER GAVE UP on my little trooper. And dare I say, he made the Terminator look like a great big sissy.

CHAPTER 2

It goes without saying that everyone on bed rest will have their own reasons for being there, different restrictions, different medical conditions and different lifestyles/tolerances, etc. but I'm going to go out on a limb and sum up the main points of the experience that I would assume would be universal.

1.   BOREDOM - The big one, the never ending one, the giant, unstoppable hemorrhoid on the ass of life. I don't care if you're someone like me who was bored in the first 30 seconds or if you're a through and through couch potato who would actually enjoy your first week or so of laying around doing nothing. Eventually, it will crawl under your skin like a rabid herd of flesh-eating termites and drive you absolutely nuts. It doesn't matter what your logical brain tells you (or the doctors, nurses, family, friends) it could be the most wonderful reason in the world for being there. For me it was, "You need to be on bed rest for the health and well being of you and your unborn child." Could there possibly be a better reason to relax and sit on my hiney for a while?? Of course not! But logic doesn't always play into situations like being incarcerated in a butt flap gown.

Just think about it on a purely sensory level:

-   you are in a hospital, out of your element.
-   you are stressed out of your mind about your unborn child.

- you are at the mercy of an ever-changing staff of strangers
- these strangers are doing uncomfortable (at best) and/or embarrassing, painful things to you every day.
- you stare at your 4 walls and ceiling all day, which will be some kind of neutral, inoffensive beige or institutional green (have I mentioned my hatred of beige yet?)
- you have windows that don't open, so no fresh air, only germy, stale, recycled air pumped up from the hospital basement.
- no ambient noise, no music in the halls, people are very quiet/hushed or sobbing hysterically.
- the pleasant aroma of rubbing alcohol and bleach and hospital food.
- the unrelenting city noise and lights all night. (though this may not be an issue for city dwellers, it only added to my frustration)
- you are locked to your bed or chair or wheelchair all day, not moving, then in your bed all night and you're expected to sleep - Helloooo??? I haven't been allowed to expend any energy all day, how can I possibly be tired?
- so, you toss and turn and have sleepless night after night with nurses (depending on your situation) coming in at all hours of the night to give you drugs or check your vitals or take your blood. My personal favorite that happened to me, "Oh don't wake up honey, I just need your arm for a blood sample!" Who in the hell can sleep through a needle being poked into their arm?? ***please read on for a more shining example of the wonderful nurses I had***

2.   LOSS OF INDEPENDENCE - as with all these categories, everyone will feel them on a different scale, but this was a real tough one for me. I have always been the one to take care of

myself and everyone else around me. I am not a control freak, but I need to at least be in the loop with anything that affects my life or the lives of those I love. I despise asking for favors or help and see it as a weakness in myself but not in others when they need my help. Messed up, I know...calling Dr. Froyd.

Anyways, when my HBR (hospitalized bed rest, aka heart breaking news) was suddenly thrust upon me, I panicked. How the hell was I going to deal with this? I went through every emotion - sadness, frustration, anger.... lots of anger, blame, fear, embarrassment, guilt, denial, hopelessness, the list went on and on. To make matters worse, most of my friends and family lived between an hour and 3 hours away. And on top of that, I was scared to tell most people (except those closest to me) what was going on because the medical staff told me several times a week that they didn't know if my baby would make it (and several times didn't know if I would make it) so I didn't want the whole world to know I was expecting. Having to tell everyone afterwards if something did go wrong, was a terrifying thought. To relive that hell over and over again was not something I was willing to risk, so I kept quiet. In hindsight I would have told the world, and accepted all the love, support and help I could but at the time I was so overwhelmed with fear I just turtled and grit my teeth.

Continuing with the loss of independence theme, I was told when to sleep, when to wake up, when to eat, when my tests were, etc. The only thing I was "allowed" to choose was when to go to the bathroom. I was informed many times that I was indeed "lucky" to have this "freedom" because many of the ladies on my floor did not have it. They referred to it as bathroom "Privileges". If I wanted to have a shower, I had to inform the nurse on duty for safety reasons. She would routinely poke her head in and ask if I was ok......there was no lock on my door. I understand the severity of my and others' situations, but I think everyone can understand the indignity of this lack of control and privacy. Especially since, in my case, I was leaking constantly the entire time I was in hospital. Not a little leak, but buckets of fluid. To the point that I was constantly dehydrated no matter how much water I drank or how many countless times I had to be hooked up to IV. I had to wear TWO of the hugest pads you've ever seen end to end 24 hours a day AND sit on a 3x3 disposable leak pad. I don't say this to gross anybody out, only to try to relay some understanding. Due to my wet situation, I obviously wanted to shower as much as possible, so I endured a lot of embarrassment. Worse than the shower humiliation, was the "pad check" every morning. I had to remove the pads every morning and lay them in the bathroom with the leak pad for the doctor and herd of students to examine every morning. Yep. Good times.

Also, I couldn't schedule visits with anyone with absolute certainty due to the obvious nature of my situation, but also due to the mountains of daily testing that was necessary which was never scheduled. Understandably, the hospital snuck us bed-resters in for testing whenever they could because, well, we weren't going anywhere! So, if a person off the street didn't show for an appointment or were late, one of us was whisked down the hall in a wheelchair to fill the spot. Considering most of us were having ultrasounds every 2 days and countless other procedures, we kept the porters very well exercised. That being said though, if a friend of mine from out of town drove all the way in to see me and 5 minutes after they got there a wheel chair showed up at my door, you can understand I was less than happy. Some of the appointments took hours so the visitor would eventually leave, and I would come back to my room to sit alone again for hours upon hours.

I was also forbidden to exercise which at the time was a huge, hairy deal. As already stated, I was a very active person. I was never a bikini model by any stretch, but always in shape. As I sat there day after day, I could literally watch and feel my muscles turning to goo. After much harassment of my doctors, they finally agreed to book a consultation with the on-staff physiotherapist for me. The poor girl showed up at my door with a "deer in the headlights" look on her face. She said, "I don't know what to do with you, you scare me! I've never had a pregnant woman on bed rest demand exercise before!" We laughed and talked and eventually I had to take what I could get. She ok'd 5 minutes every other day on a small pedal machine, only if there had been no concerns that day or the day before (which rarely happened) and I could do arm exercises with no more than 5-pound weights in my bed. Wow. Look out Mr. Olympia here comes some competition! Again, I totally understand her concern/hesitation, but I was going squirrely and needed something to do. I was allowed to walk slowly around the hallway occasionally, but usually had to wheel myself in a wheelchair. I was so frustrated and stagnant.

I didn't even have the option of choosing my own food. Hospital food has a bad rap.......for a reason. It added to the depression. The meals were nasty, luke warm and soggy and had the nutritional value of a dirty sock. Thankfully my mom visited regularly and is a wonderful cook who brought me lots of great food. The only problem with it was that all the patients shared a fridge, and everything had to be labelled and stored together. Now, from firsthand experience, pregnant women are a hungry bunch and all of us were fed the same daily rations, so I understand how the urge to steal good food would run rampant, but I was stunned how much of my stuff "went missing". I'm a generous person and very willing to share but it was like martial law in that kitchen! I even resorted to sticking humorous notes on my stuff to dissuade would be perpetrators, which did work better but not 100%.

3. FEAR - This one can encompass many things on many different levels and intensities. For me, obviously the biggest fears were centred around the wee one - Will he survive? Will he be OK if he does survive? Those 2 big ones filtered down into about 100000 smaller but still important worries. Add to that financial worries (I obviously lost my job when I got locked up), worries about my relationship that was falling apart, worries about my animals and missing them terribly, worries about all the favors and help I was forced to ask for from many people, worries about my health and deteriorating physical strength. How could I possibly be thrown back into "normal life" overnight after I'd been rotting away in there for months not being allowed to do anything but walk 5 steps to the bathroom. Let alone hopefully looking after a healthy newborn? By the end of the first month I could easily notice the muscle wasting. By the end of the second month it was painfully obvious and the simplest of movements could leave me out of breath and fatigued. Nearing the end of the third month I was basically goo. Being stagnant definitely doesn't agree with my body. Then I must go through a major abdominal surgery, heal from that, move back home (yay!), pick up where I left off with barn chores, animal chores, housework, splitting and stacking wood AND taking care of a brand-new little dude who may or may not need special care. A little daunting to say the least, especially since my partner travelled for work and was gone 8 days, then home for 6 and we lived in the middle of nowhere on a gravel road in Mennonite country. Due to my over-analytical brain and nothing to do, I thought out thousands of scenarios every day, usually not good ones.

Most days were boring and uneventful but usually at least 2-3 days/week there was some kind of stressful, terrifying event. Either the ultrasound showed something concerning (slow heart rate, lack of fetal movement, etc.) or something was happening to me (hemorrhaging, dehydration, etc.) I have never felt that level of fear in my entire life. The fear was overwhelming. It was like being thrown headfirst into a very foreign, very scary place with no escape and full of danger. I'd never felt so friggin' helpless. I was always "tough" growing up. I didn't show emotions well (except anger - man, I was good at anger!) and to be perfectly honest, I thought those that did were weak. My logic was, don't whine about a problem - suck it up and fix it. I had lived for 35 years within a very masculine energy, pushing through, goal and results oriented problem solving, swallowing any emotion that dared to raise its wimpy little head, basically I got the job done and people knew it and relied on it. Friends, family, co-workers, bosses. They all knew if they came to me with a problem or needed help, I wouldn't rest until it was done. I was referred to as people's rock and go-to person. I enjoyed helping everyone so much that I took on way too much and always put myself last because "I was tough and could handle it." So now to be thrust into this completely polar opposite role where I had to rely on other people sent my head spinning. I didn't know how to deal with it. Prime example of this was having to ask my newly retired father to drive 4 hours north to babysit all my critters every other week while my ex was away at work. During that time, he even painted the whole exterior of our house! I'm not good at delegating - I just do it. But now I had no choice. Lots of people say they've had their world turned upside down but mine got turned upside down, inside out, chewed up, spit out and thrown into a wood chipper. Even my teens and 20's motto, "Expect the worst and you'll never be disappointed." couldn't have prepared me for this.

Due to my inability to express "weakness" (fear, sadness, uncertainty, etc.) I just internalize everything, worry, feel guilty and stress. While being hospitalized I actually allowed myself to cry a few times, which is something I never did (except for Disney animal movies and SPCA commercials). I didn't know which way was up anymore. I often thought it would be easier if I had some sort of mental break because then at least I wouldn't be aware of every thought bombarding my overtaxed brain. Fortunately, or unfortunately, depending on how you look at it, I kept all my mental faculties and fought my way through.

Staying on the peri-natal floor was fear-inducing enough by itself. Every day and night you could hear someone sobbing in their room or you would hear the nurses rushing by with crash carts or whizzing someone down to surgery. And you never knew how it turned out for them because the nurses couldn't tell us for confidentiality reasons. Did the baby live? Is the mom ok? Who knows. There was lots of crying and lots of empty rooms come the next mornings. Not exactly an upbeat environment.

On a slightly more upbeat note but still related to fear, one day I heard a great big bang right outside my room. My heart damn near stopped! I got up as quick as I could and waddled to see what it was. I looked left - nothing. I looked right - nothing. I looked up - holy shit! I huge 4ft x 3ft chunk of wall had come loose and was hanging down into my doorway! It was only holding on by one corner and the wiring holding my call light/bell! I walked down to the nurse's station (too scared to use the call button!) and casually said, "Excuse me, my room is trying to kill me." They looked at me with confusion and sympathy as if to say, "She's finally lost it, poor girl!" I laughed and told them what was going on. They ran down to see and then called maintenance. What happened next was a laughable example of red tape beurocracy. A team of 8 (yes 8) people in suits and ties came up and took pictures, discussed the problems, etc. It was all I could do to keep from laughing. Then someone came in and asked if I was ok, if I'd been hurt and I had to sign a form stating I was ok. Then they put caution tape and pylons around my door and told me I'd have to stay in my room. Then maintenance guys came and removed the offending piece of wood that had been held up by GLUE! No kidding! Not a screw or nail to be found! I'm no carpenter but a huge, heavy board like that seems like it would warrant something a little stronger to secure it! Especially when it's over my head!

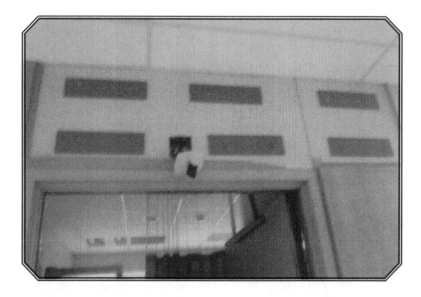

4.   Loss of Dignity - This one impacted me more than I thought it would. I think that most people (especially pregnant women) expect to have a few flushed cheeks from time to time - it's a normal part of pregnancy. I was not prepared however, for the complete and total loss of dignity and shame. My first week in and out of the emerge twice daily before being admitted was bad because each time I came in I had to meet between 2-8 people (doctors, nurses, med students, residents, etc.), go through all my history AGAIN and of course be examined AGAIN. Let me clarify that I have nothing but respect and thanks for all the medical staff that saw me through my ordeal. I understand that they were all doing their job and had my baby's health at the forefront. But now looking back (and with a healthy

awesome kid) I realize that I would have reaped huge dividends if occasionally I would have been treated like a person (who was scared and needed a reassuring hand, look or word) and not just a robotic vessel carrying a child. There were times that my sheets were ripped back, and TEAMS of people would start poking around my nether regions with the door open! I started thinking I should offer "Selfies with Stacy's hoo-ha only $1"! I was humiliated repeatedly.

Once hospitalized, the embarrassment continued on that and other levels. One incident, though funny now, blew my mind (not in a good way). I had just finished some sort of exam and was curled up in bed reeling and wanting to hide. I had a few "feeling sorry for myself" tears sneaking out when suddenly, I had an eerie feeling. Immediately, I grabbed my belly thinking something was wrong and then something caught my eye. The fucking window washer guy!! He was right outside my window going about his job while looking straight in at me! I was so shocked, I'm surprised I didn't deliver right then! Never did I think I'd have to worry about people peeking in my damn windows four floors up! I shot him a terrible look, rolled over and pouted. What if my pelvic exam had been 5 minutes later???

I swear by the time I left I'd damn near drop trou for the friggin' janitor!

CHAPTER 3

Oh joy, oh bliss, oh keep my feet from dancing.........another day of forced isolation and my butt falling asleep. This is how most of my days started. Then I would haul my butt into the bathroom and start the unending task of trying to clean myself up. Peel off wet pj's and 10lb pads and lay them out on the bathroom floor for countless doctors and nurses to examine. Freshen up as much as possible, waddle out and retrieve the soaked leak pad from the bed and add it to the pile of "examin-ables". Add yet another line to my jail-like tally I kept on my wall. Wait for the morning blood draw at 6am. Wait for what was supposed to pass as breakfast that could show up anytime between 6-8am and doctor's rounds which could be between 5-9am. Then I was ready for a busy day of sitting.

During my maximum-security lockdown, I realized that though I wasn't chained to other inmates, I was metaphorically chained to my bed and I wouldn't even be getting any cool new prison tattoos (unless you counted varicose veins and stretch marks). At least inmates get some exercise and I assume better food. They also get some socialization. This was a tough one in the hospital. I tried a few times to talk to other women on the floor, but it was so hard because the turnaround was so high and most of the patients were sad/withdrawn most of the time. They were all dealing with massive issues of their own and though for me, talking with each other would have been helpful, for a lot of them, they just wanted to be alone. It was also scary because you didn't know what their story was and when you heard the nightly emergency runs, you didn't know who it was for or what the outcome was so to go into someone's room the next day and say "Hey! How are you doing?" could be traumatic.

We had a few crazy things happen to all of us while I was there. One night during a big storm the nurses came bursting into our rooms flicking on lights and saying we needed to go out into the hallway immediately. Sleepy and confused, we made our way out only to discover that there were tornado warnings for our area and because all the rooms had such a large number of windows, we had to be in the hall with doors shut as a precaution. So now you've got dozens of high-risk pregnant ladies crammed into the hallway in the middle of the night, freaked out with all the poor nurses doing their best to move all the medical equipment, monitor everyone and prepare for a possible natural disaster. Nice. Inevitably, one lady went into labor and had to be rushed over to delivery (don't know how it turned out). The way-too-young girl beside me started flipping out and the nurses tried in vain to calm her. They ended up bringing her into one of the ultrasound rooms on the opposite side of the hall (no windows) and attempted to start an IV (I'm assuming for a sedative). It was terrible. The young girl screamed and threatened and cried. From what I could tell, they ended up having her boyfriend help restrain her and after what seemed like forever, she finally fell silent. After a few hours, the severe weather warning was lifted, and we all went back into our beds, but there was no sleeping at that point.

Another night I was awoken by screams of agony coming from a few doors down. Instinctively I crossed all my fingers and silently wished her well, hoping that this rough start would end with a healthy baby for her. It went on and on which was strange because usually at the first sign of labour, they whisked the soon to be mom away to the labour and delivery ward. It was very upsetting hearing someone in such agony for so long. Eventually, the volume of the screams faded as she was taken away. The next morning, I found out that the poor lady's appendix had burst! Poor thing! On top of everything else no less!

Warden Fetus was pretty well behaved for the first month of my prison sentence but then he started messing with me. You see, as he grew, he was pretty squashed for space - even more so than a normal baby because of my rupture. He never got to float around, he was constantly showered in amniotic fluid but never got to have a bath. He was constantly pushing against my body parts and sometimes he'd get downright pissy and have a little temper tantrum. I felt like I had a heavy weight boxer in there! I tried to console myself with the idea that he was getting a constant warm body hug, but in reality, I can't imagine he was very comfortable. He probably felt more like a pancake. Even though the nurses told me it was useless, I constantly tried to position myself with pillows and sheer determination with my pelvis or butt raised way up so gravity could keep some of the fluid inside, so he was able to move around a bit. It was really hard and usually hurt and made me lightheaded, but I kept doing it. I got many surprised looks from nurses and staff who would open my door unannounced and walk in on me in one of my inventive poses!

The Dream Team

I am thankful for all those that cared for me during my stay at the hospital - everyone from the surgeons and specialists to the porters to the housekeeping staff. But my deepest gratitude goes to a fan-flipping-tastic group of nurses. All the nurses employed there deserve huge amounts of gratitude and love and a pay raise and these special ones are definitely no exception. In fact, if I had a girl, I was going to name her after one of them. Unfortunately, due to the nature of their schedules, I only saw them sporadically, but each one of them would make an effort when they could to check on me even when they were assigned elsewhere.

The first nurse I met on the first terrifying day ended up being the first member of my team. She was compassionate, sympathetic, comforting and gentle - exactly what I needed that day. We were both around the same age and shared a deep love of animals and over the next 87 days, we developed a bond. She actually spent a couple of her breaks chatting with me about anything other than my current situation (THANK YOU). She was also the nurse on duty when I got whisked down to delivery about half way through my stay because I was having false labor (felt pretty fricken' real!). I stayed there for 24 hours all hooked up to monitors and IV's under her exceptional care until my little dude finally decided that he wasn't actually ready to come out yet (Yay!)

The second nurse was totally my type of girl. She didn't sugar coat anything, told me straight and had a great sense of humor. She shared my ability to get a little crass and sarcastic and I didn't have to worry about upsetting her. We got along wonderfully, and it was awesome to blow off steam occasionally. One night she was done her shift and was going to head home, and I wheeled past her in tears. She followed me to my room, hugged me for a long time and let me vent for a few minutes about my crumbling relationship. She stayed until I decompressed a bit and then even called back that night to check on me, on her own time (THANK YOU).

The third nurse was a stunningly beautiful young lady, with an itty-bitty waist. You would think most pregnant women would want to run her over with our wheelchairs, but she was great. She was really down to earth and seriously on the ball and smart. I felt very comfortable and secure under her care (THANK YOU).

The fourth nurse was a sweet and petite young woman with an old soul. She was a bit younger than me but embodied a very grandmotherly air about her. When she came in to do her rounds, she would never just poke, prod and take vitals and history. She would pull up a chair, hold my hand and TALK to ME, not just the body carrying a baby (THANK YOU).

I would be remiss not to mention my amazing doctor. She not only kept my baby and myself alive but her bedside manner was second to none. I only saw her about once a week due to the doctors rotating schedule, but I felt so much better as soon as she walked in the room. She is a very tall woman that carried herself in a way I can only aspire to. Probably the single most intelligent, confident, amazing, compassionate, sincere and HUMAN doctor I've ever had the privilege to be cared for by. She had a cool sense of humor that snuck by the radar of most people (especially her flock of underlings that followed her everywhere) and I looked forward to trying to catch some of it each time she visited. I couldn't possibly have asked for a better doctor. One day she entered with a new herd and wasted no time blatantly having a little fun at their expense. She came in with a militant demeanor (very unlike her) and said, "Take note!

Some of your patients will be tougher than others to handle. This one (points at me) is quite a handful. It's important to get some life history on each patient, not just medical history so you can be prepared. (students madly writing notes). What do you see? (they all look at me and my shocked face) No! Look around! (they obediently look around my room...and notice nothing, the doctor emphatically throws her arms up and sighs) She's a HORSE girl! (students notice the 1/2 dozen pictures taped on my wall of my horses) You HAVE to watch these ones! (students making notes again, oblivious to the fact they are being played) Turn your back for one second and she'll be gone! Make sure her door is shut at all times!" I am openly laughing at this point and the doctor turns to me, winks and shhh's me, eager to see how much farther she can push them! "I've seen her kick and trust me you want to be prepared for it!" At this last comment, one student looks up skeptically, followed by another and another. The doctor just smiles, and they all turn a brilliant shade of red! She pats my leg and asks if everything is ok today with me. I just smile and say I'm feeling much better now! She was AWESOME!

I also want to mention one of the heads of the NICU (neonatal intensive care unit) that I met a few weeks into my stay. I had requested to talk to one of the NICU doctors to get more information about what kind of decisions I would have to make at each stage if my baby was born early during an emergency. I dreaded hearing what she had to say, but I needed to be prepared. She stayed with me answering all my questions for over an hour. She even shared some tears when I confronted her about the horrific scenario of him being born, but not going to make it. Some of the other doctors had told me that they would just lay him on my chest and let nature take its course. I was NOT ok with this. Why would he be left to suffer?? She actually got up, shut my door, sat down and discussed the option of giving a high dose of narcotic pain control to the baby to ease his death if that was what we were faced with. I was both mortified and also relieved. Thank heavens there would be something that could be done. She added a note to my file, explaining the decision and that it was made of sound mind and for humane reasons. As she was leaving, she hugged me and recited a beautiful poem that I wish I could remember exactly, but it went something like this:

"When we step out onto the precipice, only 2 things can happen. We can find firm, solid footing or grow wings and learn to fly."

* * * * *

Luckily, about a week before he was born, I had convinced one of the other nurses to take me on a tour of the emergency surgical room. I realize this is not for everyone, but for me, preparation is everything and I really wanted her to walk me through it. She wheeled me there and showed me exactly where I would be going, and what would be happening step by step. I had lots of questions and she was happy to answer them, even though some of them surprised her. She soon found out that I was an R.V.T. and had been involved in thousands of surgeries myself. A lot of the drugs and equipment we use for animals is actually human stuff, so I was feeling much better being able to see everything. I was adamant to be awake during the c-section, but if something unforeseen came up, I wanted to know what drugs they were going to use on me. She answered with a few obvious ones and then shocked me with one - ketamine! Some of you may have heard of this as a street drug that goes by the names, special k and vitamin k and just k (and probably more, I'm not real hip to street drugs) but that wasn't the concerning part. My vet background brain was envisioning feral cats that get ketamine injected intramuscularly through live traps. They usually end up very stiff, legs stretched out, toes splayed, eyes wide and drooling!! Not exactly how I wanted my baby to see me for the first time! She laughed and assured me that would not be the case, but thankfully, I did not need any drugs and was able to avoid that possible scenario.

The big day started out normally, with no obvious concerns, but by the afternoon, things had changed - drastically. Nurse #3 was doing a daily fetal movement exam and was quickly becoming concerned. We tried having me shift positions and jiggle my belly trying to wake him up, but nothing was really working. She called for the on-call doctor and he came quickly with the ultrasound. He decided within about a minute that it was time for an emergency c-section. Holy shit. I was only at 35 weeks and 4 days. Now, I knew I had to have a c-section because he was breach, but I had been hoping for a little more notice! I got whisked back to my room for an IV to be placed (I swear my poor arms looked like a heroin addicts by that point) and yet another butt flap gown to be put on. Thankfully my best friend had just made it to the door before they took me down to surgery, so she got to come in with me (THANK YOU). As we were heading down the hall (#3 and me and a bunch of other staff I didn't even notice) Nurse #1 came running the other way. She had heard that I was coming to surgery and had actually talked another nurse into switching operating rooms with her, so she could be with me!! (THANK YOU). I felt so much better having 2 of my dream team with me I let out a huge sigh (didn't even realize I was holding my breath). They got me all set up for the epidural, which was NOT fun and then we were off to the races.

I was able to convince the anesthesiologist not to strap my arms down (THANK YOU). Not because I was claustrophobic, just because I needed to feel capable and in control of something. I was definitely capable of not moving my arms down into the surgical field. They put up the damn green drape below my chin, so I couldn't see though, much to my dismay. As the surgeon (not my doctor unfortunately) started cutting, I could definitely feel what was going on, but it didn't hurt, it was just uncomfortable and lots of pressure. As I was laying there making faces, I got elbowed in the face!!! No joke! Later, after I saw the video (you'll hear more about this in another chapter) I saw that he was pulling on me with such force, that his hand slipped off and he whacked me in the face! I was expecting a lot of pain, but I was expecting it further south!

"It's a boy!" said the doctor.

"Mama knows.... mama knows!" Annabel said softly smiling. I had "known" all along but never wanted to know officially until the big day. It's always a wonderful experience when you listen to your gut.... it's usually right.

Once my baby was out, I felt a physical relief but a mental panic. He was not crying. There was no sound except the NICU team's feet and the wheels of the incubator. That's when a few tears streamed down my face. No one would or could tell me anything. IT WAS HORRIFYING. I had to lay there for what seemed like hours while they put my insides back inside and stitched me up. When it was finally done, I thought I would get to see my baby but, no. I had to go to recovery, where I got another pleasant surprise - Nurse #4 was there! I was relieved and really hoping that all my good luck would transfer over to my baby. She took really good care of me and spent a lot of time on the phone calling NICU trying to get information for me. After another super long wait and some serious pain (I thought epidurals lasted longer......ouch) she wheeled me down to see him. I later found out that was not usually allowed while they were still working on a baby, so I was very grateful that she made it happen.

Once I got there, my heart exploded into a million pieces. there was a team of about 6 people working on him, there was monitors and medical equipment everywhere and I still couldn't see him. It was heartbreaking. Finally, one head popped up from the huddle and it was the amazing NICU doctor! She glanced over, realized it was me and mouthed, "He's ok.".

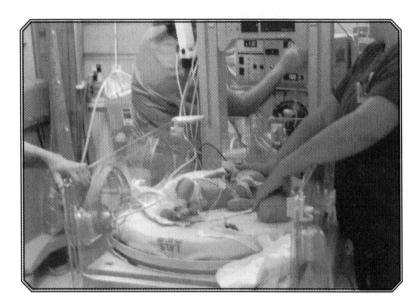

I was crying uncontrollably from a thousand different emotions at that point. They wheeled me to another small room and said they would keep me posted. Obviously, I couldn't sleep that night due to adrenaline overload, overwhelming fear, ridiculous eagerness to see him and physical pain.

When I did get to see him, I was shell shocked. He was so teeny and helpless and hooked up to all kinds of stuff. I couldn't even hold him. I could reach in and hold his hand but was not allowed to stroke him because his skin was so fragile. If I thought I had felt useless before, this was a dark new low. I had no idea how to help him and was terrified that I would inadvertently hurt him.

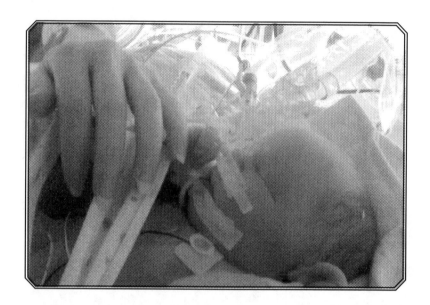

The NICU nurses were great and always fluttering in and out to check on him so I knew he was in good hands - but I wanted him in MY hands. The only thing I could do was bust ass to get him the breast milk he desperately needed. I pumped like a woman possessed. I was frustrated beyond all measure because my milk was not coming in fast enough and he needed it. He did get the small amounts of colostrum/first milk that he needed that was full of antibodies, etc. but I wanted him to get a bellyful. Finally, it did come and then we fought with latching and him being a little "lazy".

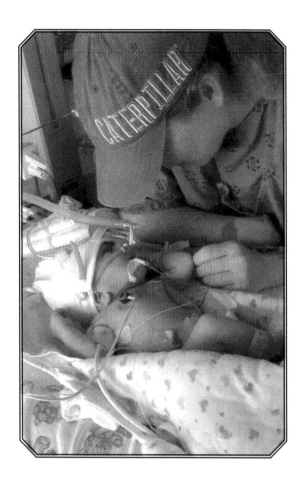

Each day he improved. They removed the ventilator. He removed the IV so many times that they stopped placing it since he was now nursing a bit. He got taken out of the incubator and put in a non-heated, non-humidity-controlled crib. I got moved from the maternity ward to the local Ronald McDonald house. Whatever you think about their food, I am so grateful for their house. It was a blessing. I was only a 10 min wheelchair ride away from him and got a real bed and a real shower with a real lock on the bathroom door! The staff was wonderful too. I stayed in the hospital for 3 days post-op and at the Ronald McDonald house 3 days. After 6 days my little trooper was ready to go! He is a tough little dude! I was so unbelievably happy to go home, there are no words to adequately express it. I was also mind-numbingly terrified. My son and I had been through hell and we'd had a round-the-clock team of doctors, nurses and specialists on call taking care of us for 93 days (87 on bed rest and an additional 6 in recovery and NICU). Now it was just us in a very remote rural place with very limited medical assistance. Out of the frying pan into the fire.

CHAPTER 4

Though there were lots of disadvantages to being so far out in the country when we arrived home, there were also many unforeseen advantages too. There were several rural programs in place to help preemies and new moms. I had a home visit nurse who came out every week at first then every two weeks for a while to check my son (weigh him, etc.) and provide me with very welcomed help, advice, suggestions. Unfortunately, one of her suggestions was to go see my nurse practitioner because she felt I was bleeding too much, too long after my surgery. I went and had an ultrasound and the floor dropped out from under me - again. They said I had a big blood clot and was not healing well and would require more surgery. I was devastated. I hadn't even healed from the c-section yet! Something told me not to give in and I went home and called my specialist. They booked me in the next week and told me not to have the surgery until they saw me and IF they deemed it necessary the surgery would be done by them. I felt better but it was still a nervous time waiting to see them. I had the ultrasound first, then saw my amazing doctor, who repeated the ultrasound right there. She was dumbfounded. What the other people had seen, apparently was my stitches and the newly forming scar tissue! She was so mad! I was floored. If I didn't have her, I would have had completely unnecessary surgery! I thanked her profusely and went home relieved. Be your own health advocate. Speak up.

I also had the benefit of a physiotherapist who came to the house to help as well because there were concerns about my sons legs due to his cramped living quarters. But probably the best visitor I got was a grandmother from an organization called Cradlelink. They set up rural moms with pre-screened, police-checked, lovely women who would volunteer 2 hours every 2 weeks in your home. They would not do babysitting or housework and you had to be home while they were there, but they provided a knowledgeable, sympathetic ear, adult companionship and the freedom to have a shower. It was a godsend. Especially when my son entered 8 1/2 weeks of colic. Yep. 8 1/2 weeks of inconsolable crying and what seemed like zero sleeping. I was a walking zombie. I tried everything. I read everything I could get my hands on, I asked everyone I knew, and I tried every trick - nothing worked. I felt like the biggest failure. I was his mom, I was supposed to be the "booboo kisser", I was supposed to make everything better. He was warm, dry, clean, fed, held and loved 24/7 and nothing helped. Quiet, dark rooms or noisy, stimulating environments - it didn't matter. Dead silence or white noise - it didn't matter. Analyzing what I ate and what he ate - it didn't matter. Swaddled or flying free - it didn't matter. He was gaining weight and doing well otherwise, so the doctors just kept saying he'd come out of it on his own. After what seemed like an infinite eternity, he did start coming out of it, but it was definitely not a happy time for anyone. The only thing that ever helped was going in the car for a drive, but I was so exhausted, I worried constantly about driving especially on the gravel back roads in the winter. Also, when he slept in the car, I obviously got no sleep and when I stopped the car he woke back up and I was on duty again without a rest. That's why I so looked forward to our visits from Chris (the helper lady assigned to us). He still cried the whole time she held him for me, but I knew he was safe, and I could actually have a shower, eat something with both hands and give my arms a break. Carrying a baby doesn't sound like much, but when you carry even a small weight for 24 hours a day it adds up especially when you are perpetually rocking, bouncing, swinging. I'm pretty sure I could have arm wrestled Lou Ferrigno and won during that time!

Out of desperation I also found a La Leche League group (breast feeding support group) in the area and jumped on the chance to hang out with other breastfeeding mothers (who I referred to affectionately as the "Boob Ladies"). They had meetings every few weeks and were helpful with advice and knowledge, but mostly I just loved the interaction and understanding. They had some extreme ideas, but I was passionate about providing my son with liquid gold (breast milk) to give him the best start possible since he had such a rough go so far. A few of us even started our own little side group which was great.

I also went to some community centre activities that were definitely not up my alley but did provide a welcome relief from my 4 walls at home. My time at the hospital and my new time at home was humongously different from my pre-baby life. I used to work ridiculous hours, volunteer regularly and have a thriving social life on top of that, but I felt like a prisoner in the hospital and now in my own home. Now, don't get me wrong, I loved that little man more than I ever thought was humanly possible and I would have gladly (and easily) kicked the shit out of a grizzly bear to protect him, but I was definitely in a whole new world.

Nobody ever tells you about the negative/darker side of having a newborn and luckily some women never experience it (bitches) but I'm here to tell you - seek people out. They are out there, you are not alone. They might not be what you think you need but you might be pleasantly surprised. You don't have to have post-partum depression to have a rough time. Sadly, my geography played a huge part in my isolation. My closest neighbours were less than desirable to say the least, especially for a first - time new mom on her own more than half the time out in the middle of nowhere. In fact, neither of them even bothered to stop in and see how we were doing or to meet my son (not that I really wanted them to though). But even in that situation I was able to find some help and I would not have made it through this time without the incredible support of my family and friends and all the wonderful people mentioned above (not the neighbours!)

My little Hulk survived the pregnancy, survived being born prematurely, survived 2 separate surgeries, and is currently kicking the crap out of asthma. He continues to amaze me every single day. It blows my mind how this little 5-pound preemie can have the heart and determination of a super hero. Whenever I'm having a bad day, I just look at him for inspiration. I hate to be repetitive but, LISTEN TO YOUR BODY. The thought of him not being here if I had listened to the specialists makes me physically nauseous. Sure, he's had some speedbumps along the way, but he is an absolutely perfect, strong, crazy, funny boy who is full of life and energy and smiles and I am so lucky and thankful that he is in my life.

87 DAYS

Part 2

Ostrich

One weekend while I was working at an animal hospital as a teenager, the vet came in (I was by myself because it was a Sunday and the clinic was closed) so I knew we had an emergency call. I asked what was up and he chuckled and asked if I had ever seen an ostrich up close. Now, this DVM was our exotics specialist but he was also a bit of a shit disturber, so I just laughed and asked what he needed me to get ready. Over the next 1/2 hour or so we proceeded to get the OR ready with fairly routine stuff (keep in mind I was an untrained teenaged kennel attendant).

Then there was a knock on the back door and he went to open it while I stayed in the treatment room waiting for the dog, cat or maybe even a lizard or bunny.... So, when a big man came through the door pulling on a horse-like lead rope I was intrigued but still expecting something like a small farm animal (sheep or goat maybe). What I was not expecting was a huge f**king ostrich! My jaw hit the floor and the doctor came in behind with a huge smile on his face.

In a display of uber-professionalism, I shook off my stunned expression and asked how I could help. The Dr had already drawn up the tranquilizer and told me to stand back. The breeder did his best to restrain the juvenile (read 6ft tall, couple hundred-pound bird) and the Dr injected it with the drugs. The next few minutes were a blur. The ostrich was NOT impressed with the poke in the bum (or wherever he got poked), slipped out of the rope and let out a screech like nothing I had ever heard before! He started running/slipping all around the room. I just about soiled my pants when it ran right at me. It was flapping its wings and squawking and had me cornered. It ran away, and I was left frozen, looking down at my jeans which had ripped straight down one thigh. To this day I still don't know if he split them with a toenail or if the fashion of the 90's had simply been stretched too far in my hurry to get away. (skin tight jeans that I pulled the zipper up with pliers)

The chaos diminished as the drugs took effect and eventually, we took control of the crazed poultry. The men were able to get the ostrich on the operating table and then the owner left. The Dr hooked it up to gas anesthetic and oxygen and my job was to squeeze the bag to breathe for the bird because placing an endotracheal tube was not an option. At this point the Dr began his attempt at a lifesaving operation to correct/relieve the bird of an impaction of food that was going to kill it. It was a long surgery and birds notoriously don't do well under anesthetic. Let alone huge flippin' ostrich's! So eventually the inevitable happened. Dr said, "shit we're losing him!" and proceeded to attempt manual heart compressions. It wasn't working so he yelled for me to breathe harder and faster for the bird.

I did my best but the mask we were using to deliver the O2 and anesthetic was not a perfect fit around the beak (obviously) not to mention we were dealing with a 4 ft long neck between delivery and lungs. So, then he yells for me to give mouth to mouth. To an ostrich. Yep. After a couple seconds of disbelief, I sucked it up and quite literally wrapped my mouth around an ostrich beak and did my best David Hasselhoff CPR! All while in complete disbelief of what was happening. This continued for several minutes until the Dr told me to stop. The bird was dead. We did absolutely everything we could. He shut off the machines, closed up the abdomen and told me to clean up while he called the owner.

The owner came back. He was acting all shifty and weird and in my naive teenage way, I figured he was just sad his bird was dead, so I was shocked to see the vets less than compassionate response to the man's request to take the body home to bury it. Normally this Dr was a warm, understanding, soft spoken man, but his hackles were up with this guy.

After a few minutes of feigned sadness, the man became increasingly irate and eventually stormed out of the clinic in a tsunami of curse words. Dr explained to me that a dead ostrich was still worth a lot of money in meat. The man put on the act of being sad, so he could sneak the body back home and butcher it and sell it, not because he wanted to bury his pet. It is both illegal and very dangerous to sell or consume meat from any animal that is full of drugs and medications.

Needless to say, that was one of the strangest and most eye-opening experiences of my entire life! I mean really, how many people do you know who have given mouth to mouth to an ostrich??!!

Chance

I learned to ride horses when I was 13 years old. I took lessons for about a year and then had the privilege of helping my coach break some yearlings (another story). I was addicted to horses and routinely talked friends and family into going to those rent-a-mule places any chance I got. There was one stable we frequented that the trails were located in a big gully/bowl surrounded by dense brush, so they were pretty confident you'd come back and not get lost, so they never sent a guide with you (not too smart on their part, but a lot of fun!)

On one trip I was given a handsome little black gelding named "Chance". When I asked the staff why he had that name, the guy smiled, then got serious and double checked with me "You're the one who can ride, right?". My confidence slowly draining I said, "Well, ummm, yes". "Good!" his smile returned "Well, we call him Chance because you got a 50/50 chance of a boring safe ride or the time of your life!". Eeeeek.

Started out pretty boring as we left the barn, he handled the steep decline to the bottom of the bowl safely, he walked patiently as my non-riding friend was trying to convince her horse to co-operate. I relaxed. My high-maintenance friend was not relaxing and not having fun. She outright refused to ride her horse anymore and was going to walk back up on foot. Not wanting the day to be over or my ride, I volunteered to bring her horse back up and bring down another. She agreed and went and sat on a stump. I took her horse, turned Chance back towards the barn and off we went. I was not expecting any trouble because rent-a-horse animals LOVE heading back to the barn. Sure enough, we made it back fine. One of the staff said they would bring down another ride in a few minutes and that I should head back down alone.

As I tried to turn Chance, he fought me a little, obviously confused and thinking he should be done for the day. After some gentle encouragement he headed off towards the steep hill. By the time I had the thought formed in my head, it was too late. It was like I was riding a totally different horse - his body language, his gait, his breathing, his energy.... uh oh.... ZOOOOOOM!!

We were off like a shot. I'm still not sure if his hooves actually touched the ground during our airborne descent down the 200-foot drop but I know they did at the bottom because when he landed, I felt my spine poke out the top of my skull and all the air flew out of my lungs. For that fraction of a second that we were still, I saw the stunned and terrified faces of my friends at the bottom of the hill. Then I saw nothing but a blur. That little shit took off at Mach 9 through the bush. The reins got caught on a tree, ripped apart and fell. Yep. No reins. I grabbed onto a fistful of whirling black mane and the horn of the saddle for dear life. That little horse was unbelievable. He was flying along those skinny trails at warp speed, ducking, diving and swerving around tree stumps, fallen logs, other riders all while squealing like a pig, tossing his head and having a grand old time!

He never once tried to buck me off, rear up, roll or scrape me off on a tree. Finally, as my luck was surely running out, he took a big jump into some deep mud and all forward movement abruptly stopped. My face met with the back of his neck (thankfully not the back of his skull) and I saw stars for a few seconds. The 2 of us stayed there for a few seconds panting, sweating, trembling and shaking. Before I had time to think, he started pushing his way through the chest deep mud slowly and calmly. He made a few attempts before he succeeded in climbing back out on the trail, shook himself off and started heading back at a walk to the base of the hill. Scared to make any sudden movements

I gently reached down and grabbed what was left of the reins while talking softly to him.

I wish that those were the days of cell phones because I would love a picture of that moment. We were quite a sight. We both had sticks and leaves in our hair, mud everywhere, cuts and scratches all over and a strangely wild but peaceful look on our faces.

My friends were just informing the staff (who had brought down the new horse) that I had flown by 10 minutes ago and they thought I was dead. The girl looked us up and down, shook her head and said, "I guess you and Chance had a hell of a ride!" I couldn't speak, I just grinned from ear to ear. Our group continued on for another hour and Chance was a perfect gentleman. On the way up the hill he was definitely tired, but he got me back up to the barn, let me hug him repeatedly and then headed off with the staff to get a bath and a nap.

Looking back, that horse should NEVER EVER EVER have been a rental but am I EVER EVER EVER glad he was!! In 30 plus years of riding, I have never enjoyed a ride as much.

Thanks Chance. For not killing me and also for the ride of my life!

Anger Issues

As a teenager, I was.... fiery, to say the least. For his entire life, my dad has been a pain in the ass in a "poke the bear" kind of way. Not a good combo. I honestly don't remember how this story started but my whole family remembers how it finished.

I was in my normal, miserable, angry-at-the-world, F-off and leave me alone mood. There was no subtlety about it. He was in his normal shit-disturbing mood and refused to leave me alone. He kept bugging me and teasing me and the madder I got the more he did it.

Finally, I could take it no more and decided to be the bigger person and walk away (high five for self-restraint teenaged me). He started to follow me. My mom warned him off. He didn't listen. I warned him off. He didn't listen.

Halfway up the stairs, he grabbed my ankle and I exploded like a rage filled volcano. I dropped to my hip, spun around and kicked him square in the throat. Yep. Kicked my father in the throat. Not his shoulder or chest - his throat. He dropped to his knees, trying to get air as I sat stunned on the stairs. I will NEVER forget what happened next. My mom (who had endured his teasing for decades) sauntered in with a dish towel in her hands, looked down at him, saw he was breathing now and said casually, "Well, she warned you." and walked away! I ran to my room and attempted to "think about what I'd done" voluntarily.

Let me state that I was not brought up in a violent household. A sarcastic, smartass one, yes but not violent. Believe it or not, we didn't even really talk about it until years later. Regardless, it was definitely a defining moment in my teen years.

Station Wagon

One of the first memorable stories happened when I was about 5 years old. My parents, grandparents, brother and I were all loaded into our station wagon (stylish) after having supper out at a restaurant. My brother and I were way in the back rear-facing seat, not wearing seatbelts (they were merely a suggestion back then). Well, we started farting around, as kids do, and I ended up with my back against the door... briefly. I do remember screaming as I fell backwards towards the pavement which was zooming past at 60km/hr. I do remember my brother (who is only 18mth older than me) grabbing my ankle. I do remember everybody screaming. But the thing I remember most of all is the face of the guy who was driving the car behind us. I swear I could bump into him 30 years from now and I'd still remember him. That poor guy must have needed to go home and change his shorts!

Physically, I was fine just a few scrapes on my hands and a sore back. My brother earned himself a gold medal from our parents and a lifetime debt of gratitude from me.

Warm and Fuzzy

A couple years out of college I took a job at a predominantly dairy vet clinic a few hours north of where I was living. Because this was in the dark ages before the internet was useful, I had to drive up there a couple times looking for a place to live. I ended up with the 2nd floor of an old house with the landlords on the first floor.

On move in day, my mom and I could both smell something but couldn't find the source. We continued with the day, cleaning, moving boxes and unpacking. Every so often we'd get a big burst of the smell and finally figured out that it stunk more when the furnace kicked on (seems obvious now but at the time we were busy and didn't notice). No big deal, we just figured that something fell down into one of the huge old cast iron grates. No problem. Just pull up a grate and have a look inside and..... PROBLEM. It could have been a dead body, an animal, garbage, I didn't know but it was gross enough to gag a maggot. Fighting the reflex to barf, I wrapped my hand in several plastic bags and bravely reached in the vent up to my elbow, half expecting to bring back my hand missing a few digits.

What I felt was warm, soft and fuzzy. Shudder. Mustering my wavering courage, I grabbed it and pulled it out. Not an animal alive or dead, but a tray of what used to be ground beef! Only now it was grey and covered with black and green fuzz and leaking a strange liquid, jelly goo. My family and I stared at each other for a while and then I headed down to get the landlord. She came up and joined in our speechless, stare-a-long. When she recovered, she dove into a string of profanity that would make a sailor blush, then apologized. She explained that the last tenants had been deadbeats who never paid their rent on time, weren't very clean or friendly and had been evicted the month prior after a big ugly fight. She said she and her husband had been surprised that they had left without incident after all the confrontation. I guess they were wrong! We ended up finding another one in a different vent as well. We cleaned everything up really well and life went on.

It was definitely a unique and memorable housewarming gift!!

Great Dane

As a kennel attendant of about 14 years old I was given a gory but necessary job one day when I showed up for work. One of the techs came up to me with a 4L jug of hydrogen peroxide and a roll of paper towels and a very sympathetic look on her face.

Turns out, that morning one of our clients Great Dane's had been euthanized. This was a Harlequin Dane (which is the big white ones with black spots that look like Holstein cows). Anyways, the owner had requested an autopsy as there had never been a definitive answer found for the poor dogs' rapid decline in health. The doctors had reportedly asked her several times if she wanted the body back afterwards to bury at home or if we were to cremate the dog. She was repulsed by the idea of taking the dogs body home, so the doctors went about the business of the autopsy.

Now, let me explain that when bodies are returned to owners, EVERY possible effort is taken to preserve the animal's appearance to lessen the trauma on the owner. Examples of this include, autopsy sutures would be as perfect, uniform and hidden under the skin as possible, ensuring the eyes are closed, bodily fluids expressed, etc. When the owner does not want the remains, the animal is still always treated with respect and dignity, but the closing of the body cavity is done quickly and practically and with large, external, functional stitches and the body is not cleaned up or made esthetically pleasing.

This is where I came in. The owner had called back and changed her mind about bringing the dogs body back home. Obviously, this was a terribly sad and traumatic day for her, so everyone understood her change of heart. Keep in mind, however, that this is about a 160lb, mostly white dog who had already been in the freezer for about 7 hours (euthanized animal bodies are kept in freezers until the cremation company comes to pick them up). Due to its size, they had laid it on its back with the 4 legs in the air, the eyes were frozen open, the jowls were all hanging upside down and open and the chest and abdomen were covered with frozen blood. After my monumental job of cleaning the poor critter up, the doctors were going to be replacing the sutures.

I attempted reaching in to clean him but due to my only being 5'2" this proved next to impossible. So, I climbed in. Yep. One of the techs came back about an hour later to find me sweating and straddling a huge dead dog in a chest freezer, surrounded by about a dozen rolls of blood-soaked paper towels. She could barely control herself as she told me that they had just received a phone call from the owner saying she had changed her mind AGAIN and now she didn't want the dog back anymore! So, I hauled my aching back and shoulders and my frozen feet out of the freezer. I still felt compassion for the lady and the dog but man, I really earned my stripes that day!

Amusement Parks

As kids, my friend and I used to go to a popular amusement park every summer. The summer when we were 12 was the most memorable one. We were rollercoaster junkies and that year we got to go 2 times, once at the end of the school year on a class trip and once on our own later.

On the school trip a bunch of us raced to the big coaster and I ended up paired with the shortest girl in the class. Who cares right? Wrong. Apparently, she should have measured herself beside the "you must be this tall" sign. Now, this coaster was old school and only had the hand rail to hold on to (no body harness). As we were climbing the first hill she started crying. I did my best to comfort her but kept telling her to hold on tight. During the first 1/3 of our descent, her rear end lifted up a few inches off the seat and her eyes damn near popped out of her head. Holy shit. By the time we reached the bottom, she was laying down at my feet sobbing and clutching my ankles for dear life. I would like to say that I helped her get down there, but I honestly don't know - everything happened so fast. Whether it was her, me, us, gravity, dumb luck - who cares, because she was a hell of a lot safer down there than flying in the air! When the damn thing finally came to a stop she was in shock and pretty banged up, but otherwise ok and alive. The staff of the park and our teacher rushed in and took over. We wished her well and took off to ride coasters all day long.......the beauty of the invincible mentality of the young!

Later that summer my friend (not the short one) and I returned to the same amusement park (with no sense of impending doom I might add). We went on ride after ride and were having a blast. Then we went on our favorite coaster (not the one from the previous story) for the 3rd time that day. As we were heading up the first hill there was a lot of screeching and clunking, enough so that we took notice. I poked my head over the side and saw that our car was off the track. No shit. It was still attached to the car in front and behind but had shifted off the rail and was kind of being dragged. Well, to say we freaked out was an understatement. We started yelling, screaming and waving at the quickly disappearing staff - who waved back.... thanks. The guy behind us told us (very rudely) to shut up and sit down. To which I replied (very rudely) what was happening and specifically what he could do with his big mouth. Then he checks over the side and starts yelling and waving.

So, we're at the top of the hill. My friend and I look at each other, hold on with all the strength of professional arm wrestlers and take a big breath (possibly our last). Thankfully this coaster had a lap bar so we delusionally felt a little safer. During our short and dramatic ride, all the people on the platform became aware of what was going on due to the spectacular pyrotechnics show from all the sparks flying off the wheels. By the time we stopped there was quite a few staff and one dude in a suit waiting for us. They were all over us asking if we were ok. In classic adrenaline soaked teenage style, we said we were fine and ran off to get on another ride!

In hindsight, I'm pretty sure we could have at least scored some free passes for life, since they were probably thinking they were going to get sued........damn adolescent brain!

Annabel and Sebastian

The first time I met Annabel was in 2003. I was on a job interview at a humane society and while I waited in the lobby for my appointment, I noticed a little head poking over the reception desk repeatedly. She soon asked where I had worked, and we got to chatting and discovered that we had bumped into each other several times in the past at several different clinics. We hit it off right away in a way I've never experienced before. It was literally like I already knew her, we flowed like an old married couple right out of the gate!

After my interview with the boss at the humane society, or the Devil's Wingman as I came to call her (oh the stories I could tell...) I ended up with the job and I started in 2 weeks. Great! Except I lived an hour and a half away and my roommate was getting married in just under 2 weeks and I was in the wedding party! Needless to say, that the next 14 days were a whirlwind and thank heavens for Diane (again) because she lived 1/2way between and let me rent a room off her until I found a new place.

Day one of my new job as head of the animal health department was busy, as any first day usually is but I got to see the funniest damn thing that completely broke the ice and made me feel right at home, courtesy of Annabel. I was making the rounds, checking on all the critters in the morning before we opened and when I walked in to the main cat room, I heard her talking to someone, so I didn't say anything. Seconds later, I realized that she was talking to herself (warning), she was actually giving herself a pep talk. I felt a little bad for staying silent but honestly could not stop listening, it was so intense! She was psyching herself up to touch a 3-pound rabbit who was giving her attitude. "OK Annabel, you can do this. It's OK, it's just a little rabbit. Come on!". Once I discovered what the pep talk was for,

I couldn't contain myself any longer and burst out laughing. She spun around wide eyed with a lovely crimson hue rushing up her face. While wiping tears from my eyes I walked over, scooped the little heathen up and put him in the fresh cage she had prepared. By this time, she was laughing too, and we had cemented our friendship (being saved from a savage beast has a tendency to do that....).

Our friendship blossomed, and I soon met her husband and the three of us hung out a lot. They were easily the coolest and craziest people I had ever met. Their attitudes and exuberance for life were contagious. They were also the most outwardly loving people I had ever encountered, which was very difficult to get used to for me. I have never been a hugger, I have always liked my 3-foot bubble of personal space, but these guys burst through my bubble with total obliviousness and joy and would giggle at my discomfort (with no ill intent). They always say "I love you" at the end of phone calls and when parting and it took me years to return the words (though the sentiment was always there). I always used to tell them that they meant so much to me I'd give them a kidney if they needed it but was not comfortable saying "I love you". Come to think of it, I had past boyfriends who complained of my lack of ability to show emotion.... Anyways, the kidney thing stuck and for years I would say and write "kidneys" in place of "love" while talking to them or in birthday cards, etc.

We had many adventures together, but some of my favorites are below.

*   *   *   *   *

One of the first trips we took together was a road trip to Tennessee to visit the Jack Daniels Distillery. Sebastian and I were both die hard JD fans and Annabel was always up for anything. With the invincibility of 20-somethings we all went to work for the day on a Friday, then left directly after work and drove straight through all the way to Tennessee. We traded off for the driving, but all stayed awake the whole time. It was insane. We were hysterical and sleep deprived. By the time we got to sleep for the first time, we had been awake for 42 hours! We stopped at a gas station about an hour out from our destination and they went in the store for supplies, but I stayed outside and leaned my forearms on the car with my head down trying to stretch and find my 9th wind. A local guy walked up near me and said (in a huge southern drawl), "Honey pie you don't look so good!" I laughed and told him we were going to the JD factory and how far we'd come. He looked stunned and said, "Shit girl! I've lived 'round here my whole damn life and I ain't never even been to the whiskey factory! Y'all are crazy!" He certainly hit that nail right on the head!

From there we drove on, navigating our way through the small towns and then almost had an accident. There was a big billboard that said in bold print, "Alcoholics, there's help ahead." That was fine, but I shit you not, the very next billboard said, "Jack Daniel's Next Right"!! We laughed so hard that we missed the turn off and almost drove off the road!

We stopped at a little mom & pop restaurant for breakfast to kill some time until JD opened, and I had a small meltdown. I'm one of those people who once I start laughing, I CAN NOT stop. I turn bright red, tears stream down my face and I don't make any noise. The silliest thing can bring this tornado of hysteria on (especially after being awake so long) and it's impossible to stop. As I was sitting across from these two nut jobs reading the menu, they started having a very serious discussion as to the difference between tater tots and tater babies. I listened for a minute then felt the impending lunacy creeping up on me fast. I lost it. They looked at me confused as to why I was laughing. Herein lies the next problem. While losing it, I am incapable of speaking and the mere mention of the subject or questions about it will send me over the edge. Once they realized what was going on, they intentionally started teasing me and trying to push me over said edge - thanks guys! Of course, this is when the waitress came over to take our order and gave me a look that was fear mixed with annoyance. I'm sure she (and the other patrons) thought I was high as a kite. Annabel and Sebastian didn't skip a beat and proceeded to inquire at length about the size, shape, consistency and taste of the tater tots and tater babies. I was done. I couldn't breathe, I couldn't see through my tears and I was starting to get dizzy from lack of oxygen. They had to order for me. I finally calmed down after what seemed like forever, ate my food and left a BIG tip! I still don't know if they ordered me tots or babies, but I was sure glad to get the hell out of there!

We headed over to the factory and had the best time. They give long, informative, super cool tours and you get to see the whole place which is beautiful and surrounded by nature. They still do a lot of things the old-fashioned way and you feel like you've gone back in time. Even if you don't like to drink JD (what's wrong with you??) I'd still highly recommend the tour, it's awesome. We stayed there most of the day and spent way too much at the different gift/souvenir stores. They had the coolest stuff and if we had the room, we would have come home with a lot more than T-shirts. They had everything you could imagine made of the old whiskey barrels, some serious one of a kind stuff. The only let down of the whole visit was that Lynchburg is a dry county. So, you're at the Jack Daniel's factory and can't even buy a drink!

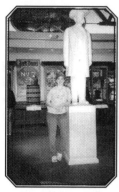
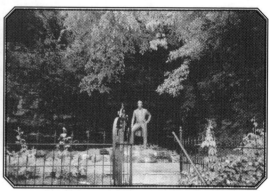

My boyfriend
Jack and I

The man, the legend

After leaving there we still had a several hour drive to Kentucky to meet up with Sebastian's rock-climbing friends. We were staying at a small, climbers only foothold up in the mountains. Annabel and I don't climb but we carried some gear and tried to look the part. We set up tents and I managed to stay awake for about 1/2 hour before collapsing and sleeping like a hibernating grizzly bear until the next morning.

*   *   *   *   *

I'm going to start this story by saying that I am a very proud Canadian. I love my country and I am very thankful to live here. That being said, I was absolutely stunned several years back when the province of Ontario made the mind-numbingly stupid decision to ban pit bulls. I was horrified. I was embarrassed. I was confused and saddened. Ontario is an incredibly diverse place to live and the fact that the government was enforcing such a racist, ridiculous policy was completely archaic and, pardon me, balls-to-the-wall fucking stupid! (sometimes I'm not clear about my emotions, so let me know if I'm being too subtle......:) I mean, banning an entire breed because of a few isolated incidents is crazy! That would be like packing up all the men in the world and shipping them off to an island and killing the ones who stayed because a few of them are class A assholes (who I usually end up dating!) The only difference being that the men have the choice to be an asshole whereas the dogs have no say in what environment they are forced into or the training (or lack of) they are exposed to.

Anyways, Annabel's friend was putting together some fundraisers to aid in the fight against this stupidity and try to advocate for the pit bulls. We jumped on board right away. One of the activities was a charity bowling tournament so we signed up and raised as much money as we could. Annabel had the great idea to dress up and come up with a team name. Normally I'm not a flamboyant person but was willing to do anything to try and put a stop to this so I agreed. When I showed up at her house that morning and saw the box of goodies, all I could do was shake my head. Our team name was "The Stinky Pits" and we all had puffy glitter glue emblazoned T-shirts stating just that. She had also bought lots of hair clips with beads, feathers, sparkly doo-dads and some bracelets. The piece de resistance though, was 8-inch-long, clip in hair extensions which we were to attach to the armpits of our shirts for effect. You do what you gotta do - I donned my gear and the Stinky Pits went out and bowled our asses off. Unfortunately, the government proceeded with its insanity and those of us on the front lines had to clean up their mess for years to come. Exhausting resources trying to ship dogs out of the province, continually bugging other shelters to take our pits, boarding pits while their owners tried relocating and sadly in the end being forced to euthanize way too many. I always wished that the beurocrats would man-up and come and witness firsthand the heart wrenching sorrow of a family euthanizing a beloved pet or the grief and stress of shelter staff euthanizing entire litters of puppies just because of their breed. Maybe a good slap in the face of reality would make them think twice about putting their John Hancock on a law. Just as a side note I would like to point out that I've been working in animal hospitals and shelters for 3 decades and I would trust any pit bull, Staffordshire, Mastiff, Doberman, Rottweiler WAY more than a small or toy breed dog - those little buggers offer to bite 100 times more often than the big fellas. Anyways, I'm starting to rant. The point of this story was the "Stinky Pits" and I so wish I had a picture to share with you, we were quite a sight!

*   *   *   *

Among the many things Anabel and Sebastian opened my eyes to was the amazing experience of travel and the insanity of the work, work, work, save, save, save mentality I was stuck in. What was I saving FOR if I never did anything with the money?! Hmmmm...they might have a point here. I have always been frugal (read tight) with my hard-earned dough and the thought of frivolous spending makes my stomach turn. I don't shop, I don't care about clothes (I shop at thrift stores) or jewellery and I take care of my stuff, so it lasts. My only guilty pleasure is concerts. So, after some serious effort on their part, they actually convinced me to go to Jamaica twice and I will be forever in their debt! I had no idea how much I needed to relax until I got there!

When you get to Jamaica it's like time literally slows down and your blood pressure and heart rate are cut in half as soon as you get your first big breath of that beautiful ocean air. It's awesome. Now, in classic A+S style, we didn't stay at a fancy resort, we stayed in a cottage far from the main tourist areas on the edge of a cliff not a beach. It was amazing. Not everybody's cup of tea but it was absolutely perfect for us. They had been to the same place the year before, so they knew the owners, our specifically requested taxi driver (Eltado aka Dave), his friend (Rasta Robbie aka The Colonel) a local guy (Andrew) and a small boat captain

(Vincent). The welcome we received was awesome. I've never felt so instantly comfortable with strangers before. It's an entirely different experience to travel with the locals, and we had immeasurable fun! The other benefit was that the other locals and vendors didn't harass us at all when we were with these guys.

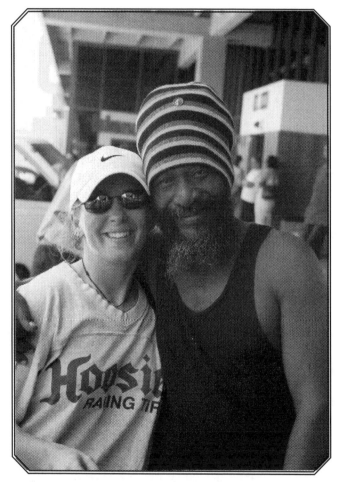

Rasta Robbie and I

Right beside our cottage was a fabulous vegetarian outdoor restaurant called Just Natural, run by a special lady named

Theresa. The food was rid-ic-u-lous! We ate there at least once a day but usually more. Somehow a fruit smoothie tastes 100 times better when it's made with fruit that's literally been picked within the hour and you're sitting in the Jamaican sun with your best friends!

The only "touristy" things we did were go to the local market and take a bus to Margaritaville.

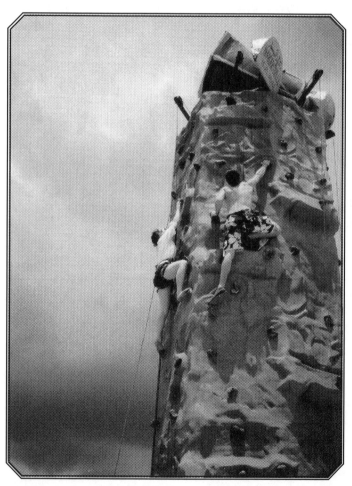

Bottomless rum punch and rock climbing – smart!

The rest of the time we spent with the guys and swimming/ floating in the pool or the ocean. It was a very steep decline on a rickety staircase to get down to the ocean, but there was a large flat rock at the bottom big enough for 2 lounge chairs. Once you jumped in, the water was immediately about 20 feet deep and you were surrounded by open ocean on one side and jagged rocks on the other - not for the faint of heart.

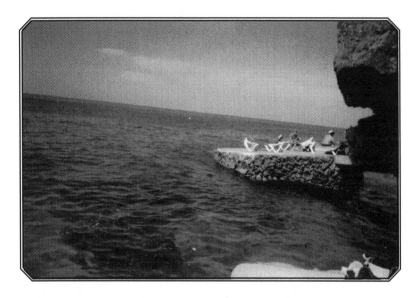

We snorkeled every day and saw some cool stuff. Annabel even got to meet a fish close up that tried to leap over her head and ended up tail slapping her on the face! We never thought of the danger and had a great time. Sebastian even went night diving with Andrew. Night diving! Annabel and I stayed on dry land and I tried my best to calm her down while on the inside, both of us were panicking. Occasionally you could see their flashlights underwater but for the most part we just stared at the black water hoping he'd survive. In thanks for our worrying, the boys threw a large lobster up on the small rock at our feet and scared the crap out of us. It's only been in the last few years that I've really realized how insanely lucky we all were to avoid drowning, being injured and avoiding sharks and other dangerous critters.

More stories about this crazy pair are peppered throughout this book and about a thousand more in my head and heart. They are truly one (two) of a kind!

Legs Up

I was very eager and full of beans when I started my first RVT job out of college. I worked whatever hours they wanted me to and I took on lots of extra duties. One of these "extras" really stuck in my memory and the memories of some random strangers.

The clinic I worked at was a mixed animal practice (farm animal and house pet) and we had been working with a farmer who had an unknown illness going through his barn. His cattle were getting quite sick and not responding well to treatments we had tried so far. My boss had been on the phone with some colleagues and they had all decided that it would be worth the farmer's money to send one of the animals for a post mortem (autopsy) at the veterinary college. My boss called the farmer to let him know what the next step would be in our hunt for an answer and he was pleasantly surprised when the man told him, "Well you're in luck, one died last night!"

I continued on with my morning duties, not paying much attention to the conversation just being happy that we were finally going to get this poor guy some answers. My boss approached me a little while later and said he had a special job for me. I was excited and curious as to what it could be and when he revealed that I was going on a road trip today I was thrilled. I loved getting out and doing something different. He said I would be driving the carcass to the university, which was about 2 hours away. I was bummed because I had to tell him that I had never driven with anything as big as a livestock trailer and he reassured me there was no problem because it was a relatively small steer that fit in the back of the farmers pick up truck. Great news! I got ready to leave because the farmer was already on his way in. When he got there, my jaw dropped

The truck was like something out of bad sitcom. I had never seen anything in such bad shape before. Every piece of the exterior was a different colour because it had come off a different vehicle at some point. It had NO rear-view mirrors of any kind. The front bumper was LITERALLY held on with baler twine. There was a huge crack going across most of the front windshield. But the worst part was the dead steer in the bed of the pickup. He was bigger than expected and was causing the truck to tilt. He was in full rigor mortis and was frozen solid as well – with his 4 legs straight up in the air! My boss and I stood there in shock for a few minutes taking in the whole scene then the 3 of us scooted back inside to warm up (it was the dead of winter). I was the first to voice my concerns, and I had several. My boss backed me up on most of them especially the road-worthiness of this vehicle and the visual state of the steer. The farmer said he didn't have a big enough tarp to cover the animal and that he had put it in his old farm truck because he never thought it would be going on such a drive. He also told me to dress warm because there was a leak in it somewhere and the exhaust fumes got into the cab, so I had to drive with the windows open! It was approximately minus 20 degrees. With the invincibility of youth, I laughed and grabbed the keys from him. I borrowed a couple sweaters from the receptionist, got a huge fuzzy blanket for my dog (who used to come to work with me) and off we went.

The ride was surprisingly uneventful while driving through the countryside, but things sure changed when I entered the city limits. The veterinary college is pretty much smack right in the centre of Guelph which is a not a small place. It is a very busy city since on top of its normal population it is home to thousands of students. Additionally, I showed up there right at lunch time. Not great timing for a subtle entrance.

At first all I noticed was a few strange looks from passing motorists but when I had to stop at traffic lights things got more interesting. Pedestrians would point and shout and laugh. Drivers would stare in disbelief at the Jed Clampett truck with its unusual cargo. I even had a lady who was walking 3 dogs almost lose control of them when they saw/smelled us coming. The funniest though was a tiny little elderly lady who was riding passenger in a car beside me and was literally dry heaving, then looking back at the steer, then dry heaving again! Stop looking!

I had one scare when I took a corner a little too quickly (in my hurry to be done with this experience) and the steer rolled off his back onto his side. The whole truck bounced and there was a terrible bang when he landed. Even my poor dog jumped and whimpered looking around frantically at the dilapidated truck.

I made it to the college, they unloaded the beast without incident and we were back on our way. I've been on many road trips, I've been on many crop tours and I've been in many crappy vehicles but none of them could hold a candle to this experience!

Tonsils

I struggled with tonsillitis my entire childhood. I would get it every couple of months, get thrown on constant rounds of antibiotics and feel pretty crappy. I never understood why no one would take them out and after years of torment, I was finally referred to a "specialist" (I use the term very loosely) at 18 years old.

He was a pompous little prick obviously suffering from Napoleon complex and had the bedside manner of a cockroach, but I was desperate. See, I was starting college in a few months and really wanted the offending little organs removed before getting there. He agreed to do it early in the summer and swore that I'd be back on my feet in about a week, plenty of time before college.

The day of the surgery came, and I was a little nervous but more excited to be done with my damn tonsils. I knew I would be sore afterwards, but it couldn't be too much worse than years of repeat tonsillitis, right? Ha! When I woke up, the heavy-duty drugs were still working so I felt pretty good. As they wore off and the real pain set in, I was still ok. Once I got home, I expected a rough first night and I did have one. The next day, I felt terrible and the pain was escalating rapidly regardless of pain medication. I went to bed that night and was soon awoken by the need to vomit - great, that will be fun. Once poised over the sink, I realized that I didn't need to vomit stomach contents, I needed to gag up copious amounts of blood clots lodged in my throat. Disgusting and more than just a little worrisome due to the sheer volume of them. Off to emerge we go. Luckily/unluckily Dr Dingbat was on call. He came in not even trying to hide his annoyance at being called in, yanked my head back, pulled down my chin (ouch) and started poking around without a word to me. I shoved his hand back and tried to speak but he cut me off saying there were some "bleeders" that he needed to cauterize....ummm....I'm awake you maniac! He said it wouldn't be too bad and to suck it up. In hindsight at this point, I should have kicked him away from me and headed out the door, but hey, it's 20/20, right? He proceeded to climb down my freshly chopped up throat and chemically cauterize me with silver nitrate sticks. Between the pain, the gagging, the taste and the ever-leaking blood I damn near barfed on his shoes (wish I would have!) He finished, told me to get some sleep and left. I toughed it out for the next few weeks and when I had to go back in for my recheck and complained about still being in pain and still occasionally yakking up blood, he told me I was a slow healer and I would be fine. What was supposed to take about a week ended up taking 3 months.

The first sore throat I got at college was a doozy. I literally felt like someone had jabbed an ice pick into the right side of my neck. Like I said, I've had lots of sore throats, but nothing like this so I went to a walk-in clinic. The doctor there looked down my throat and said, "Oh you've just had your tonsils out...". I informed her that the surgery had been done months ago. She stopped her exam, looked at me and then grabbed a pen and asked me lots of questions. She wanted to know who did it, what I was told about the results, etc. She proceeded to inform me that my throat was "butchered" and the reason for the intense localized pain was that a small piece of the tonsil had been left in! The other side had been dug out so aggressively that I actually had a crater as opposed to smooth tissue! (to this day, if I don't chew popcorn well enough it will often get stuck in that pocket and I have to make very unladylike sounds and push on my neck to dislodge it). Anyways, she said I should get a second opinion from another specialist and get it fixed but after the hell I'd been through the past 3 months I declined. She said she was going to alert the doctors governing body about the surgeon and his mess. She gave me some meds to deal with my current situation, I thanked her and left.

I never had to see Dr Dingdong again but have heard many stories (none good) about him through the years. How do you become a specialist if you suck at what you do and none of your patients are happy??? I finally understood why no one wanted me to take my tonsils out as a kid.

The Cruise Missile

As a young teenager I was lucky enough to learn how to ride horses. I had a great coach who taught me the basics and threw me in headfirst. Her knowledge and my unbridled love, passion and respect for horses led me to develop a comfort level and talent for riding. I never had the desire to show or compete, I just loved being around horses, being in the barn and experiencing them on every level. Their power, strength, stamina, gracefulness and heart, their movement, their smell, their responsiveness. I loved trying to figure them out and how to successfully communicate with them through body language, cues and patience. I loved the barn environment - the soft sounds of horses breathing, munching hay, the smell of the hay, the leather and the horses. It always had a glorious calming effect on me no matter what mood my teenage brain was in.

I learned how to ride on two horses that were polar opposites from each other. A 3 yr old Quarter horse named "Dimples" who was a big, strong, powerful mare full of energy and spirit. And "JJ" a sweet old broodmare who had seen it all and done it all. By riding both simultaneously I learned very quickly.

The barn had many boarders and I was quickly honored to be asked to exercise other people's horses for them while they were away. Dream come true! I would ride anything, anytime anyone would let me. A $35000 push-button, beautiful gelding. A regal, immensely tall thoroughbred cross that took some getting used to because of his long strides and the fact that he only rode in English tack and I only rode in western or bareback. A little Quarter horse shit disturber who like to bite. The list went on and on. I went to a few shows where I was the gopher and warm-up/cool-down rider for my coach and her friends. I was so happy!

Then I got the ultimate pat on the back when my coach told me I could help her break a couple of two-year olds. I was over the moon! "Poncho" was a sweet, laid back gelding and "Cruise" was a powerhouse, spitfire mare. I was a sponge soaking up all my coach's knowledge, watching her with Cruise. I was getting very attached to Poncho and little wary of Cruise (first horse ever). She was a force to be reckoned with. Coach did 99% of the work with her and they were amazing to watch.

After several months, I started working more with Cruise, but it was never the same as being around any of the other horses. You could never let your guard down and she didn't enjoy any "soft" attention (speaking to her, grooming her, petting/ scratching her). I respected the hell out of her and I'm thankful for my experience with her because she taught me a lot. She brought a lot of qualities to the forefront that her more laid-back counterparts did not.

One sunny summer day, coach looked at me, smiled and said, "Today you're going to lope Cruise." Being young and indestructible (and dumb) I jumped at the challenge and felt so proud that coach thought I could handle it. Poncho and I had been loping smoothly for quite a while and I had been watching the other pair very closely. I was a little nervous but mostly excited. I did all the ground work with her - grooming, tacking up, lunging and was feeling confident. I jumped up on her and we took it slow for several minutes to get used to each other. She was great! It was an awesome feeling sitting on this powder keg and feeling the enormity of her engine. Unlike any other horse I'd been on. We went through the motions - walk, jog, patterns, whoa, back up - all with great success. Cruise was breathing hard, we were both sweating, and I was grinning from ear to ear. Coach gave me the nod. On the next trip around the arena as we headed towards the corner, I cued her with my leg and a kiss sound (universal cue for a horse to pick up the pace). She was NOT impressed. She tossed her head, danced around and snorted. Disappointed, but not about to give up, I tried again. She responded by some fancy crow hops, tossing her head and slamming on the brakes. Stunned but still upright I looked at coach. She told me I definitely had to get a few loping strides out of her and then she would get on. Setting the precedent that this dangerous behaviour was going to get her out of working and listening was not in the cards, so I set my jaw and tried again. You know how hindsight is 20/20? Well....attempt #3 went down in the history books. I wish there were cell phones back then that could take movies because I would love to have documentation on what happened next.

I asked for a lope. She told me in no uncertain terms to "F off". There was crow hops, cow kicks, rearing, snorting, head tossing. Then she proceeded to buck while somehow serpentining her spine a couple times which unseated me. Then she bucked with a power that was out of this world. As I was coming down from this last buck, I landed square on her rump and she was already on her way back up again. She propelled me into the air with the force of a rocket ship. I soared through the air for what seemed like minutes until I hit the barn wall. Then I fell to the arena floor with a thud. Just in time to see 2 cement-hard hooves hurtling towards my face at the speed of light. Thank heavens I froze with fear because if I'd moved an inch, I would have been dead. Her hooves went on either side of my head and one actually ripped out a small chunk of my hair on the left side.

She took off around the arena squealing like a pig, bucking and farting in some sort of victory lap. Coach ran to me to ask if I was ok and then went to catch the poltergeist horse. At this point I realized the wind had been knocked out of me and I hadn't breathed in a while! Coughing and gasping I got some air and started my body scan to see if I was in one piece. Who knows how, but I was ok. I was banged up, bruised and scraped but nothing broken. I got up slowly and looked over at coach and Cruise. The horse was lathered up (thick, frothy horse sweat) and breathing hard but had an air of calmness about her. Coach's eyes were still wide, and she didn't say anything. I walked/limped over, climbed back on and coach led us around the arena once. Then Cruise and I went around at a walk once. I stopped her, backed her up, stopped her again, then climbed off and handed the reins to coach and sat down in the dirt. I stayed there for a long time as coach cooled off and put Cruise away. When she came back, she squatted down and said, "Great job getting back on kid!" then "Holy Shit that was insane!" We rehashed the experience from both perspectives. Hers from watching the mêlée and mine from being bounced around like a pinball. This story is the opposite views combined into as cohesive a read as possible.

I never did ride Cruise again, but I will always remember what she taught me.

Poncho

Poncho on the other hand was the sweetest, most laid-back fella I'd ever met. Nothing fazed him. The biggest issue we had was lighting a fire under his butt to keep him moving! He was awesome, and I was in love. Logically I knew he wasn't mine of course, but my heart liked to pretend he was. He would follow me around the barn like a dog, he was a real joy to ride, he was perfect.

Once he had a minor injury to his front right hoof, so the vet had said not to ride him for about a week. No problem. I spent my time loving him up, grooming him and puttering around. The next day I came out, expecting more of the same, but I got a huge surprise. Not a good one.

The barn owner stopped me on my way in the and threw his arm around my shoulders.

"Why don't you ride Poncho tonight dear?"

"I can't he's hurt."

"Just walk him around, he'll be fine."

"But...." I was confused.

"Sorry kid, I sold him. He leaves in 2 days." and with that he turned away and scooted back to the safety of his house where he wouldn't have to witness a young girl's heart being broken for the first time.

I was devastated. I loved that horse more than anything in the world. I went into his stall, hugged his beautiful neck and cried for a long time. Sweet bugger tolerated me and just kept eating. I brushed him with a slow, appreciative reverence that night. Tacked him up and brought him to the arena for the last time. Usually it was a very busy place in the evening, but it was strangely empty that night (thankfully). We walked around a couple times, then he started to limp slightly, so I jumped off. I hung out with him for about another hour, hugged and kissed him about a thousand times and eventually closed the stall door and walked away broken-hearted. I cried all the way home and when I got there, I lashed out and tore a strip off my parents for not buying him first. Then I ran to my room and stayed there for hours. Ridiculous, I know but I was a hormonal teenager who had just lost my first love, logic had no place here.

I didn't go back to the barn for a couple weeks. During that time, I stopped wanting to run over the barn owner with a semi truck. I knew all along that Poncho was his horse and that one day he'd be sold. That was the man's business. I guess in my delusional happiness, I had chosen to deny that reality. At the time I had wished I'd known earlier but looking back, having the Band-Aid ripped off quick was better. The next time I talked to the barn owner he thanked me repeatedly for all the work and time I'd put into Poncho because it helped immensely with his end price. I took the compliment but fought back tears again because to me it was never work to be with Poncho.

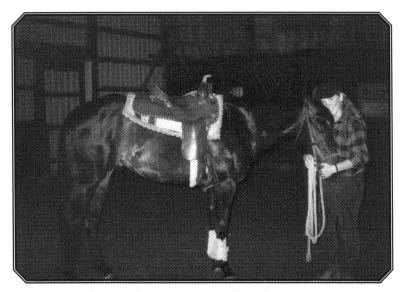

My sweet, sweet Poncho

I've ridden tons of horses since those early days and I've never met one like him. I hope whoever bought him loved him at least half as much as I did.

Excuse Me...

Just like most of the stories from "back in the day", this one still leaves me shaking my head.

We were at an outdoor BBQ/bonfire at my friend's farm house and there was probably about 20 people sitting around, chatting, enjoying a few beverages and swatting mosquitoes. I was regaling the person sitting beside me with a riveting tale and having a great time. During my conversation I felt a tiny tap on my shoulder and I turned to see an even tinier lady beside me that said something so quietly I couldn't hear her. I smiled, held up my index finger and said, "Just a second please" and turned back to my initial conversation. We were neck-deep into it again when I felt another teeny tiny tap on my shoulder. I turned and said, "Sorry, I'll be right with you, I'm almost done!" and proceeded to get lost in my conversation yet again. Please keep 2 things in mind: 1. I love telling stories (can you tell??) 2. I was three sheets to the wind. The next tap I felt was more forceful and the lady had actually stood up and was leaning over me and my wobbly lawn chair. Geez! I thought, how about some patience?? As I shot her a less than pleasant look, she pointed at the ground and barely above a whisper said, "Excuse me, but your shoe is on fire!"

After a millisecond of stunned silence, I looked down and what do you know, my foot really was on fire! I jumped up and stomped my shoe on the grass. Luckily, my shoe was extinguished, unluckily, it made a gross gooey mess on the ground and stunk to high heaven. The stunned quiet of the crowd soon burst into a roar of laughter once they realized everything was ok. Needless to say, that was a very sobering moment!

In our inebriated state, which clearly qualified us to play detective, we decided that my shoe had simply gotten too close to the fire and because it was a running shoe, the thick tread (or possibly the beer) prevented me from feeling the heat.

In the end no one got hurt, we all had a good laugh and learned a lesson and the new girl got many lectures on how sometimes its ok to break the bonds of propriety and just yell, "Holy shit! You're on fire!"

Brownies

Lots of kids have memorable experiences from Brownies/Girl Guides or Beavers/Cub Scouts and I was no different. At about 5 years old my Brownie group went on a weekend camping trip. I was excited and a little apprehensive but 3 of my best friends were going too, so mostly excited. We did a lot of the typical stuff you'd expect but we also did one extra. We all had to take turns cleaning the outhouse. Probably not the best idea for a bunch of 5-year olds. Especially since the outhouse was literally that - a wood shed with no running water and a plastic toilet seat bolted onto a piece of plywood. We didn't know enough to question it at the time (Hey! Hindsight! How you doin'?)

By the second day I felt pretty crappy. The leaders kept telling me I was just homesick and to go have fun - until I started vomiting. Then I was whisked away into the leaders' cabin which had a full bathroom, complete with toilet, sink and shower. They set me up on one of their beds and rejoined the others. I spent the day scared, alone and fighting off the war raging in my stomach and intestinal tract. They did check on me periodically and replenish my cup of water but that was it. I was miserable and wanted to go home.

When camp was finally over the next day, my parents came and got me and took me right to the hospital (I can only imagine the words they had with the leaders). Now, comforted to be back with my folks, but terrified to be at the hospital, I was not a happy camper (pun intended). After several hours the diagnosis came in - E. Coli poisoning. Great. I got admitted to the hospital for several days in the kids' ward. Out of all the bad stuff that was happening the one thing I was grateful for was the IV fluids. After just one bag ran into me, I felt a lot better and tried to convince everyone I could go home. It didn't work.

The first couple days/nights were a blur of vomiting and diarrhea and fear but on the 3rd night things got worse. Nurse "Evil Witch" showed up for work and unfortunately for me she was assigned to "care" for me. I remember waking up with a throat and mouthful of vomit which of course found its way out all over my sheets. I buzzed the nurse and did my best to clean up a little. She came in like a drill sergeant with PMS, whipped my door open, flipped on the lights and emphatically showed her disgust. She started ripping off all the bedclothes (while I was still in bed) while berating me for not making it to the bathroom sink. She vented for what seemed like forever and I just wanted to hide. I felt horrible. She slammed a large plastic bowl on the freshly made bed beside me and said, "THAT is for vomit!" and she stormed out slamming the door. I stayed awake that whole night too scared to fall asleep in case I had to barf again.

By the time my parents came back in the next morning, I must have looked terrible. I briefly told them about Lucifer's nurse and my dad disappeared for a while. I don't know what he said or what happened, but I never saw that nurse again.

I recovered after a few more days but have never been the same since. My guts were permanently damaged, and I have struggled with GI issues ever since. If your cousin's boyfriend's great aunt's garbage man has a stomach bug - I'll get it. If I eat anything other than my tried and true menu of benign food, I pay dearly.

Anyways, the point of this story is this - if you are unhappy at your job or you find that it just doesn't suit you - LEAVE!! Afraid of fire? Don't be a fireman. Hate animals? Don't be a vet. Are you mean and cruel and intentionally horrible with children? Don't work on the f'n children's ward!! (my public service message for the day).

I have mad respect and love and appreciation for nurses and the insanely wonderful work they do. This rotten apple certainly didn't measure up and is in no way a reflection of the amazing nurses busting their asses to take care of our broken asses every day.

Sheep

One of the first surgeries I was able to take part in was a sheep C-section back in my early kennel attendant days back in the late 80's/early 90's (timeline will be important later).

The large animal vet had brought the sheep back to the clinic to perform the surgery, a luxury he wasn't frequently able to do due to the size of most of his patients. She was anesthetized and prepped for surgery and away they went. I was kept busy fetching various medication, equipment and towels and getting a bird's eye view when I wasn't on a gopher run.

Suddenly, 2 little squirming lambs were out, and one was shoved in my arms. I wrapped it up in a warm towel and zoned right out in a state of bliss. I sat on the floor cradling this little miracle until the mom was recovered enough to have her babies returned to her. Then I started the huge task of cleaning the mess, which wasn't even a big deal in my stunned, happy state. Everything went great, mom and babies were healthy, farmer was happy, Dr and techs did a great job and I was over the moon. I barely remembered on my way home to stop at the bank (long before the days of interact). I walked in and waited my turn in line. I noticed that the person ahead of me stepped away as far as the congested line would allow. I wasn't offended because I knew I smelled pretty strongly of sheep.

Once I got to the teller and started talking to her, I watched her eyes widen and her body lean back. Confused, I continued on with my request. She quickly gave me my money and I left. As I walked out to my car, I wondered what was going on, so I checked in the car's vanity mirror when I got in. Then I laughed and laughed and laughed! Stuck onto one of my ridiculously large 80's hoop earring was a substantial glob of something birth-related and next to it in my light brown hair was a large blood stain! No wonder everyone was avoiding me! And why the hell didn't anyone call the cops?? If I saw someone walking around with blood and guts all over them, I'm pretty sure I'd do something about it!

Shelter

While working at a shelter out west, I had a few memorable experiences. It was a very small shelter that serviced a huge geographical area and had very little public support at the time. It was also smack dab in the middle of a massive feral cat population. Unfortunately, due to the immense size of that population vs. the small size of the shelter and severely restricted funding, most of the wild cats were put down. This job sadly landed in my lap. We had a never-ending intake of these poor, sick, usually pregnant wild cats that the city workers and some locals brought in in live traps. Literally dozens each and every day. They were terrified and unable to be socialized and put into homes. It was heartbreaking but a far nicer way to go than starving to death, being hit by a car, dying of some horrible disease in the street or being eaten by a coyote, dog or bear.

One time I got a hard and fast reminder to not be lulled into a routine with these guys (which was easy to do because there were so many and most of them were too scared to move when I gave them a gentle poke of sedative through the cage. There was a small calico cat balled up at one end of the trap and as my assistant maneuvered the trap so I could get better access, the cat went ballistic (picture the Tazmanian devil in a cage). There was urine and feces spraying everywhere and somehow the door opened. The cat flew out of the cage and without thinking I reached out and caught it by the scruff of the neck. I quickly dropped the needle and grabbed its back feet, trying to restrain it and get it back in the cage. Problem was though that she was small, had very little scruff to hold onto and was completely nuts by this point. She was able to free her head, spin it around and bite me twice in the meat of my hand below my thumb. Bad enough, but on the second bite she didn't let go, just held onto my flesh like a dog with a tug toy, her teeth imbedded fully up to her gums. In a lot of pain but seizing the opportunity to get her contained while she was preoccupied biting me, I shoved her and my hand into another cage and she let go of me. My helper was completely shell shocked and staring at me with wide eyes and an open mouth. My adrenaline had allowed me to handle the situation and ignore most of the pain but now that things were settling down the pain was increasing rapidly.

I took stock of my injuries – I had 8 perfect puncture wounds, 4 on the top of my hand and a matching set on my palm (4 canine teeth x 2 separate bites), my forearm looked like Freddy Krueger had his way with me from all the deep scratches that her 10 razor sharp claws of her front feet had assaulted me with and I was bleeding steadily from all the wounds. My grey uniform was well spattered with blood and my hand had already swollen up to twice its normal size. I grabbed a clean towel to wrap my arm with and told my helper to get me to a hospital asap. Cat bites can be very dangerous due to the bacteria they have in their mouths and the depth of their punctures (cat scratch fever, etc.).

We showed up and the triage nurse just looked at my blood soaked SPCA clothes and towel and simply asked, "cat or dog?". I answered "cat" and she immediately took me right in. I was given IV antibiotics, cleaned up and sent home with 2 prescriptions of more antibiotics.   The next couple of weeks were very painful and awkward because she had ravaged my right hand and arm and I'm right handed. I held nothing against the poor cat, it wasn't her fault she was just in survival mode. Interesting though because I've been working in vet clinics for 3 decades and this was my only cat bite ever - but it was a doozy!

This story that didn't end well for either of us is a good reminder to everyone to spay and neuter your pets. If you don't want them or can't care for them anymore, please don't just let them go. Find a new home or shelter or even humanely euthanize them – it's a lot better than life on the streets. It's crazy how fast they can multiply in the wild. In just a few short years it is estimated that one female cat and her offspring can produce thousands and thousands more offspring!

*   *   *   *   *

Another story from that shelter was not for the faint of heart but interesting none the less. As I said, we serviced a huge area and had ridiculously poor funding and massive quantities of animals coming through the door. Now, in most areas, all animal remains are sent to a crematorium to be disposed of. In this area however, they did not have that option because it was simply not available and on top of that, even if it was, they could not afford it. So, the only answer they had was to use the local garbage dump which was obviously not ideal for so many reasons but was literally their only option.

There is literally no such thing as a regular quitting time at a shelter and you get used to staying late quite frequently which is why it surprised me that the staff was very strict about the dump run time every day. When I asked why, I was informed that the dump insisted that our vans be there before 3:00pm or we would be turned away. Confused, I inquired again as to the logic of this (knowing the dump stayed open until 6:00pm). The dump insisted on having all the animal remains there by 3:00 because they needed to be sure they would have enough garbage come in afterwards to bury them deep enough that the bears who scavenged there wouldn't be able to dig them up and eat them! Apparently in the past when the bears had done so, they became affected by the sedatives in the euthanized animals and acted drunk and lost their fear of people. Definitely a potentially very dangerous situation that I never would have thought of!

Teens

So many stories from my drunken, stupid teenage years, but there's a few that definitely stick out in the ol' memory.

1.   My best friend and I were at a keg party having a really good time. She and I were sitting on the floor going through a bunch of cassette tapes figuring out what to put in the stereo next (yes, young ones, we used to have to physically change the album!). A guy across the room yelled "Hey!" trying to get another guys attention and naturally we looked up. Mistake. He proceeded to flick/snap a beer cap trying to hit his buddy. Mistake. His drunken aim was way off and as my friend looked up, it hit her in the face. She doubled over screaming. I thought it was a bit of an overreaction until she looked up at me. The white of her eye was rapidly filling with bright red blood. She looked like something out of a horror movie. The weirdest thing was that it wasn't dripping out on her face. Instant sobriety. We ran to the bathroom to assess the situation. Obviously, she needed a Dr, but we were hesitant. Her and I were supposed to be at each other's house, our boyfriends and the rest of the party goers were leery because they had served us as minors. Finally, I convinced the most sober guy to drive us to the hospital. He dropped us at the door and took off. Thanks.

I went into the emergency ward with her, got her registered and they took her right in. Now came the fun part - I had to call her parents from the pay phone in the lobby. As my nervous fingers dialed the phone, I glanced at the clock on the wall. It's noticeable ticking seemed to be counting down to my impending doom. Had this been a minor UPI (unexplainable party incident) we would have brushed it off, made up a lame excuse and moved on. But a bleeding eyeball warranted a little more action!

Ring ring, "..........Hello?"

"Mrs. Smith Tina's OK but we're at the hospital and we need you to come!"

"I'm on my way!"

It was 2am. Oh crap. We're in trouble. I figured after this all panned out her and I would be grounded until our mid thirties. Her parents got there in record time. They glared at me with Lucifer-like intensity as they strode past me and disappeared into the exam room. I waited for what seemed like a really long time, then a nurse came out and told me Tina would be staying overnight, no, I couldn't see her, and I should go home. Luckily, the party had chilled out and there were some mostly sober volunteers to come get me.

The good news was that the beer cap had cut her eye a few millimeters below her pupil, so she didn't lose her sight. She ended up with a pretty interesting scar through her iris but was none the worse for wear after healing. The moral of the story?? Come on say it with me!! IT'S ONLY FUN TIL SOMEONE LOSES AN EYE!

*   *   *   *   *

2.   At another party, this time out at a cottage near the lake, I was the one who got the shit end of the stick. At some point in the night, I had decided it would be a good idea to take off my shoes (who says booze affects good judgement??). As I stumbled around outside, I failed to spot a smashed beer bottle and proceeded to step on it. Son of a bee-otch that hurt!

I hollered, and a couple guys scooped me up and brought me inside. I left a trail of blood on the floor all the way to the couch (what do you know - alcohol really does thin out your blood!). Good news - there was a nurse there. Yay! Bad news - she was hammered. Boo.

There was a large triangle shaped piece of glass in the arch of my right foot and she was at least "with it" enough not to pull it out until she had gathered some supplies. By supplies, I mean a dish towel and a 1/2 empty bottle of vodka that had been pushed into a frozen watermelon to make slushies. Good enough! She doused my foot with vodka. Wow. That was not pleasant. Then she told 2 guys to hold me still while she pulled out the glass. I gritted my teeth. She counted down....3..2....1....oops! Oops??? WTF?? Well, she only got about 2/3 of the big chunk out but the top broke off in my foot. Fan-fucking-tastic. Oh well, in my classic teenage invincibility mode I said screw it, we bandaged my foot with a t-shirt and duct tape and we continued on with the night.

The next morning my foot was swollen and so friggin' sore. Instead of seeking medical attention, I fabricated some stupid story and tried to ignore the throbbing (great plan). To this day, I have to walk up stairs on the ball of my right foot because if I step on the edge of the stair with my arch I'll drop like a bag of hammers!

I swear to you that I graduated elementary, high school and college all with Honors. Though I can see how that would be very hard to believe........

*   *   *   *   *

3.   Some of the guys knew of a secluded beach cove about 20 minutes from town. It was great, very shallow, gently sloping sand (not rocks), was usually warm, had a small piece of dry land big enough for a bonfire, 20 odd people and a bunch of coolers.

The only downside was that to get to it you had to climb down a 100-foot cliff on a pretty precarious path that made its way down to the beach. No problem, we were young and immortal. We were also lucky because no one ever got seriously hurt. Especially given the amount of alcohol involved and the fact that it was usually pitch black. We went there regularly, and the place was given the moniker, "The Badlands".

One night, everything was going along great and everyone was having a blast. Most of the group was wading out in the shallow water. A highly intelligent move since we were all drunk and the only light was from the piddly little bonfire that was having trouble staying lit in the breeze and was about 150 feet away.

Gradually, the rowdy conversation started dropping off and there was a brief moment of eerie silence before we all screamed/yelled/swore and started running towards the beach. Well, running may be generous. Do you know how hard it is to run in waist deep water, while drunk, in the dark without spilling your beer??

Once safely on dry land, we were all talking at once trying to figure out what happened. One of the guys climbed back up the cliff and shined a huge floodlight from his truck. We all saw a large moving black mass out in the water. You see, we had all run like scared little kids because we had felt a bunch of slimy things bumping against our legs. And now to see the size of the school we were stunned. We didn't know what kind of sea life had just crashed out party but we sure as hell stayed on dry land for the rest of the night. Even in our present state, it just didn't seem like they were harmless little guppies. There was something very unsettling about the situation. No harm, no foul, the party continued. Later on that week though, there was some interesting information on the news.

Apparently, there had been a barge that dumped its ballast water in the lake and it was full of some type of eels that were not native to our area. These eels had multiplied like crazy, quite enjoying their new habitat and had now become the target of the Fish and Wildlife guys to get under control. They had to warn the public because these particular eels, though not venomous or electric were still large enough to give a hell of a bite!

Like I said, I can't be sure what critters we encountered, but the creepiness, the sliminess and the timing all point in one direction - EELS! Thank heavens none of us got bitten, we lucked out again. We did continue going there to party, but no one was real keen on getting in the water anymore (at least we smartened up a little bit!). That experience always makes me laugh because it is so like a cheesy bad horror movie. Dark night, drunken teenagers being eaten by scary possessed eels! Classic!

Tattoo

Even though I thought I was incredibly stealthy and covert as a kid/teen, I discovered it was pretty flippin' difficult to pull one over on the old man. Even my genius brother who had the charisma, brains and talent had a tough time fooling the old bugger.

When I was 15 I did it! It took a couple weeks of planning and the help of my accomplices (mom and brother) but I did it. My friends and I went to a carnival/fair in the states where there was a booth that applied incredibly real looking temporary tattoos. We were planning on going back to the fair one more time before it ended, and thus, my idea had taken root. I explained my idea and we figured out the script and were all eagerly looking forward to ink day.

To put it mildly, let's just say that dad is 3 million percent against tattoo's, especially on his teenage daughter. I had been interested in tats since about the age of 12 and we had several debates about them. He was quite volatile about it. In his opinion (which is usually the only one that matters!) the only people that got tattoos were military men, bikers and inmates. This was going to be good. To make it even better, he had booked family portraits at Sears the day after I was going to get it -Halleluiah!

My biggest fear was not being able to keep a straight face and blowing the whole thing, but I was determined to try. That old guy had been tormenting people for years with practical jokes, teasing, etc and he was way overdue for some serious payback. We went to the fair. I got a black rose with blood dripping off it right below my collarbone. The guy who applied it made me want to bathe in Purell, but who cares, it was on! I came home and headed upstairs to where my mom was doing her hair for the pictures. I showed her, and she took a minute to prepare herself, then gave quite a performance (loud enough for him to hear). I stormed out on cue and went to my room. My brother jumped in with perfect dramatic timing complaining about unfair sibling treatment and suggesting appropriate punishments. Dad said nothing. WTF? Did he figure us out? Ha! Nope! He was so ridiculously angry he chose to ignore the situation until the pictures were done and would "deal with me later". Good news - it was working better than I thought. Bad news - I had to keep a straight face even longer. Thankfully, I had a lot of practice at being scowly and silent so that's what I did. I imagine it was harder for my brother because he was generally pretty happy, but his acting chops would help him out.

Somehow, we made it through the pictures and got back home with palpable tension mounting. I was directed to sit in the sunroom and the others were shoed away into the kitchen. Then I sat through the world's longest "I'm so disappointed in you" speech of all time. As if it wasn't hard enough to keep a straight face, my accomplices had snuck behind him in the kitchen and were laughing silently. He finally asked to see it and as I shifted my collar, I knew I was on the verge of losing control, so I said quite loudly, "FINE. If you hate it so much, I'll just go wash it off!". He stared at me for about 5 seconds in disbelief. Then I started laughing hysterically and ran for my life! I made it out of the house and halfway down the street before he gave up the chase. Thankfully my youth and genuine fear for my life had given me some extra speed.

I cautiously made my way back home after about 1/2 hour not sure what to expect. Luckily, because I shared the blame with 2 other people it wasn't too bad. To his credit, he said something no one ever thought we'd hear, "OK, OK you got me!". Chalk one up for the kid!

During my 20's and 30's I got several large REAL tattoos which I managed to keep hidden from the old guy until I was 39. That big reveal was also planned with accomplices - my sister in law, 2 young nephews and my 3-year-old son. Being in front of his 3 grandkids helped to keep his reaction G rated this time. Plus the fact that the tats are all far more tasteful than the blood soaked rose and the fact that I was pushing 40 instead of being too young to drive probably helped too!

Snakes

During business hours one day at the vet clinic there was a lot of excitement and the staff were all talking and wound up when I got there. I had no idea what was going on and before I had time to ask, 2 of the male vets came into the treatment room struggling to carry a large metal trunk about 4ft x 3ft x 2ft. Everyone gathered around (me included) and watched intently while they opened the latches.

Surprise! Two huge snakes! Everybody was amazed, and questions started flying. We soon found out that they were boa constrictors and that due to our proximity to the US/Canadian border we were the vet clinic selected for any animal seizure by the border guards.

Apparently, there was some American strippers that were trying to cross the border with several hundred pounds of snakes crammed into a relatively small trunk. The border guards didn't like the accommodations (and rightly so) so we got the job of assessing the animals for humane reasons (yay for the border guards!)

The 2 snakes were docile (thankfully) but each required several people to handle them. The smaller one was dealt with first to be measured, weighed, examined, etc, which took half a dozen staff. Then the big one was pulled out and I was elated to be asked to help with his exam. My job was to use a soft broom (I'm serious) to push down behind his head and keep me safely out of teeth range while the others stretched him out for measurements.

I was thrilled, excited, blown away by the sheer size, strength and beauty of this animal. I was leaning all my weight on this broom and though he was slightly subdued the snake had no problem moving me and the rest of the team around with very little effort. He was gorgeous. Later I found out that he was close to 15 ft long and a couple hundred pounds.

Luckily for him and the other snake they were both deemed in great physical condition (borderline chubby) and the only concern was their travelling conditions and work environment. They were eventually returned to their owner.

It still blows my mind though, how a 105lb female entertainer could have handled and used these snakes in her act all by herself. We had a hell of a time with a whole team! Mind you, I couldn't hang upside down on a pole either, so maybe veterinary professionals are just a weak breed??

Border Crossing

I grew up in Sarnia, Ontario, Canada. It is a mid-sized city (about 70 000) located on the Canadian/USA border, separated by the St. Clair River and Lake Huron and connected by the Bluewater Bridge.

As a teenager, my crew made many trips across the bridge - long before the new heightened security of today. Worst case scenario you might have to show your birth certificate, but most times we were just waved through. We would go over for essentials like cheaper gas and booze. A car full of us would head over, fill up the tank, then head to the liquor store and fill up on supplies to get tanked. We would bring back ridiculous amounts of booze, get the older guys to claim 2 bottles and head on our merry way. There were even times where some of us would literally be sitting on mickeys of liquor (one under each thigh). Definitely not intelligent, but back then it was no big deal.

We did get pulled into the secondary search once on our way over and we were a little concerned but not too worried because we had nothing to hide yet. They split us up and started questioning us separately. We were a rough looking bunch but I'm pretty sure it was just a scare tactic. We were dumb but not dumb enough to carry anything illegal or bring any buddies who had lost border crossing privileges. The officer who questioned me was definitely trying to make some kind of point and it was hard to keep my teenaged f- you attitude in check. He started ripping apart my purse and laying everything on the counter between us. He asked me about EVERYTHING. He examined each stick of gum, unscrewed a pen I had, opened a couple of sealed tampons (???), then pulled out a small bottle of aerosol hairspray and set it on the table with great flourish and looked at me. I was very confused. He asked what it was for. Was this a trick question?? I pointed to my hairspray helmet head (the 80's do). He looked very doubtful and attempted to find the secret trap door in it. I said as calmly and non-sarcastically as I could that he should be careful or else it would explode. After he broke the spray nozzle off, he finally put it aside to delve deeper into my purse. He then found a Q-tip and held it about an inch from my nose while asking what it was for. Seriously??? I mean it's not like it was a crack pipe for heaven's sake! I took a deep breath and explained to him that it was for removing "Coop". That is what we used to call it when your eyeliner would run/smear down from your eye a bit and you would look like Alice Cooper. One of the guards behind my interrogator muffled a chuckle and my guy was visibly embarrassed. He gruffly told me to collect my stuff and go wait for my friends. I couldn't help myself from saying, "OK thanks, but you can keep the broken hairspray it's no good to me now." We ended up all being cleared, and we went home with lots of similar stories. I am thankful for the work the border guards do to keep us safe (especially now a days) but I really think this was a bit overkill. I mean really, you'd have to be a hell of a MacGyver to rig up a weapon out of a tampon, hairspray and a Q-tip!!

Another story which paints the guards in a far better light happened when my girlfriend and I went over with her boyfriend to get some automotive part for his van and have lunch. This guy used to be called "Creeping Jesus" because he looked just like him and he prized his van so much that he would drive slowly so he didn't get it dirty or chip the paint. It was one of those vans like the A-team with a solid back (no windows). He had it done up like crazy - bright red paint job, carpet inside, seats all removed from the back, custom lights inside, custom stereo, etc. Anyways, we pull up and the guard notices me in the back as he's questioning the other 2. He immediately walks around to the back door, opens it and stared at me with an intensity I still haven't forgotten. He never took his eyes from mine and said very slowly and very seriously, "Young lady, DO YOU WANT TO BE HERE?" I was shocked at first and then realized what this scenario might look like. I smiled warmly at him and said very sincerely, "Thank you. Yes, I want to be here. This is my best friend and this is her boyfriend. I am OK, thank you again". He nodded and closed the door. Even in my teenaged brain fog, I was very thankful that there were guards like him looking out for people.

The best border experience I had by far was in the late 90's. My friend and I were moving back to Ontario after spending a year in British Columbia. We had driven through the US for part of the trip and were crossing the Bluewater Bridge to come back into Canada. Our cars were packed to the rafters. There was not an ounce of space left. I could only see out about 2/3 of my front window and my driver's side window and nothing else (probably illegal?). So, we pull up to the booth and I got a very young officer who was puffing out his chest and shining his mirrored Magnum PI sunglasses......oh goody, this should go well. Sure enough, he was a dick. He took one look at my overstuffed car, snickered and asked me if I had any booze. I kind of laughed and said that there was a 1/2 bottle of whiskey buried somewhere in the trunk (I've been told that sometimes I'm too honest). He smiled, pulled his shades down to the tip of his nose and said, "I'm sure they'll find it in secondary." He gave me a search slip and pointed. I started vibrating and said, "Come on! Seriously?" He gave me an icy look and pointed more firmly. It was all I could do not to throttle the little over compensating wiener. We had been in the car for days, we were 5 min from home and this asshole was going to get my whole car ripped apart! (FYI for those that don't know, nobody helps you put your car back together after a search). I was close to tears of frustration. I pulled in, parked and got out of my car to wait. The douche bag pulled my friend in behind me and we commiserated with each other. Then a female guard headed over to us and when she was about 10 feet away, she paused and said, "Stace? Holy crap is that you?" I didn't skip a beat, and headed over to her all smiles, saying things like, "Wow! Great to see you! How have you been?". We chatted for a minute and I explained what had happened with her fellow officer. She scoffed and said he was indeed a dick. She also said that there was no need to empty the cars, just open the doors and trunk and she would do a half assed visual search and we could be on our way. Grateful to our core, we happily obliged, scooping up the odd thing that fell out when we opened them. We thanked her repeatedly and headed off. To this day, I still have no idea who she was, but I sure am glad she knew me!!

Kyle Calving

During and after college I worked at a dairy research facility milking, feeding, calving and doing the grunt work for the researchers (blood work, feed trials, etc). Hands down, I worked for the best guys. They teased me mercilessly, worked me tirelessly and I loved every minute of it. The camaraderie in that barn was like nothing I'd ever been part of before or since at a job.

I was on call for calvings one night and sure enough, the night security guard called me just after midnight. I drove in, in my sleep deprived state and assessed the situation. It was a first-time heifer (potential for a hard pull) but she looked ok at the moment, so I assembled all my gear and called my boyfriend to say I'd be awhile. The security guard wanted no part of watching or assisting and the other staff were all busy at a livestock show out of town, so I was crossing my fingers for an easy pull.

No such luck. Big bull calf + first time pelvis = traffic jam. The heifer and I gave it our best try for about 15 minutes with little progress, that big bugger was digging his heels in. So, I called the vet - who was busy at another calving and said he'd be there as soon as he could (read too late). So, I called my boyfriend back and just said, "Come quick I need you!" and hung up. You see, this fella was the most squeamish person I'd ever met. So, if I said WHY I needed help, he never would have shown up. To his credit, he came fast but didn't want to come past the door. He caught sight of me covered in birth secretions, surrounded by calving equipment and he headed back out gagging. I yelled for him to come around the side of the barn (thankfully her birthing stall was right next to the side door). He did as I asked but wouldn't look in. Of course, I knew how difficult this was going to be, but I had no other choice. While waiting for him to get there I had devised a fool proof plan (because those usually work out for me, right?). I tried explaining it to him, but he didn't understand so I just said, "Turn around, back in here and do as I say" (First time a guy ever listened to that) Being the trooper he was, he did just that.

The calf was in the right position, with front legs and nose visible so I attached the calving chains around his legs. Then I placed the calving jack under mom's rump and directed my backwards, blind assistant to the pole and crank handle. "All you have to do is pump the handle until I tell you different." I said. You could see the colour draining from his face and all the hard swallows he was making but he toughed it out. I helped mom and guided the calf and he was the muscle. Every time she would moan or move or fart, he'd freeze up and I'd try to start talking about some benign topic to help take his poor mind off what was going on behind him. We were all doing great, front end, shoulders, chest and abdomen were all out, calf was alive, mom was ok, and the boyfriend was still upright and breathing. We were just waiting on mom for one more big push and him for one last big pull .... here we go!

What happened next was like slow motion. The calf fell out into my arms and we both went down onto the bedding (he was huge!). The calving jack clattered to the floor. Mom continued the last of her big push. I looked up and saw a huge glob of fluid/blood/goo/lubricant launch out of her backside and sail through the air. Meanwhile, my trusty assistant was straightening up now that the pressure was off the jack. You know where this is going don't you? Yep. He got hit in the back of the neck by airborne cow birthing fluids. There was actually a "smack" sound when it made contact. Some slid into the T-shirt, but most fell on the ground. I sat in stunned silence under the wet clumsy calf. I couldn't make out any of the words he was saying except, "Oh

F**k! Oh F**k! Oh F**k!" as he danced around swatting madly at his neck/back. He looked like he was being attacked by a swarm of bees. He ripped off his shirt and ran out of the barn, jumped in his car and left! I burst out in laughter and continued on with mom and baby. It took me another hour or so to finish up, clean up and make sure junior and mom were doing well. I found his abandoned T-shirt in the parking lot. As I headed home, I could just imagine the damage control I was going to have to do, but I just couldn't stop laughing. You couldn't have planned that if you tried!

Surprisingly, he was a great sport about it. I think after he showered the goo off, the awareness that he helped save one and possibly two lives softened the blow a little. But I did have to hear about it for a couple years after the fact!

In the end, it all turned out great. Mom and baby did fantastic, boyfriend survived, I got a good laugh, and you got a story! Many thanks to my backwards assistant.

Meeting the Parents

So, you know how nervous you get when you have to meet a significant others parents? And you know how after the initial meet and greet you feel a relief that it's over and maybe a little stressed after seeing the gene pool first hand? Or maybe it actually wasn't as bad as you expected? Well, this isn't one of those times.

I was dating a guy in college and it came time to meet his folks. So, I'm all wound up and getting more stressed out the closer we get to their house. He keeps assuring me that his parents will love me, and everything will work out fine - famous last words.

We pull in the driveway and see his dad heading for chores, so we make a pit stop and I met him first. He's lovely. A big, statuesque man with a soft voice who refers to me as "Dear" several times. I'm relieved and actually enjoyed talking to him. Then he says he has work to do but will be in soon. Now my stress returns as we start heading towards the farm house to meet his mom.

We got in the door and barely got our shoes off when this little bundle came hustling down the hall. She was a very short, very round little woman full of energy. She ignored her son, walked right up to me, smiled, grabbed me by the shoulders, looked me up and down, smiled again stated warmly, "Well hi!" I naively started to relax, then she continued. "Well you certainly won't have any trouble popping my grandkids out of THOSE hips!!"

I don't know whose jaw hit the ground first, mine or my boyfriends, but he collected himself first and started to tear a strip off good ol' mom. She was shocked and held her hand to her chest and said she meant it as a compliment! WTF?????

If anyone can explain to me how that can be a compliment, please let me know! Especially since at the time I was in the best physical shape of my life, with an athletic build, 21 years old and maybe weighing 120 pounds!

For the rest of the evening she acted as if nothing had happened. I did my best to forget about it and make it through the night, but you can be damn sure I made sure she wasn't behind me when I bent over to put my shoes back on when it was time to go!

Baby Chicks

While working at the dairy barn, I was asked to help out a co-worker to unload a shipment of baby chicks at his farm on my lunch break. Several of us went over to help after we finished the morning chores. I had never done this before, but I was definitely looking forward to seeing the teeny little fluffy dudes.

The transport truck was already there and in position beside the barn. I followed the guys inside and awaited the impending cuteness. As I was handed my first flat of peeping, adorable-ness I was momentarily stunned. I don't know how many of them fit on each tray (approx 2 1/2 feet square) but it was enough sweetness to require some insulin. One of the guys hollered at me to "Get moving! There's 10 000 more out here just as cute!" I snapped out of my sugar-coma and asked what to do with them. I was told to start unloading them over in the far corner. Off I went, knelt down and started picking the little dudes up one by one and placing them on the straw bedding. I was almost done emptying my tray when I was startled by a loud burst of laughter from all the guys. Tentatively, I turned around to find myself surrounded by a sea of fluffy yellow chicks about 15 ft deep. The guys were busting a gut.

"But how...?" I asked. In response my boss grabbed a tray of chicks, walked over and tipped them out from waist high! Gasp! The poor little buggers! Suppressing the urge to swat the guys, I hurried over to make sure the chicks were ok. Slowly, I started to realize that the little fluff balls hardly weigh anything at all and they were landing/bouncing on a freshly chopped, thick, soft bed of straw. They were completely fine. OK lesson learned. Score 1 for the boys.

We finished unloading the truck with me being exponentially faster and more helpful. (Though I never did tip them from waist high, I always squatted down and gently tipped them out). I took A LOT of heat for that day for a long time!

Externship

Like most college kids, I was always eager for the next challenge, event, experience and usually jumped in head first, brain second. When it came time for my class to pick a location for our externship in senior year (1-month placement in the field) I was stoked. All I cared about was finding a cool new place to explore that had a large animal clinic. I gave no thought to any other "minor" details like where to live, how far away it was, how inconvenient it was regarding weather, travel...etc. On the whole list of clinics that were accepting us, there were only 2 offering livestock exposure - one of which was in my hometown. Well that would be far too intelligent a choice! Staying with the folks for free, using their car, already having worked at that clinic for 5 years.... the list goes on. Nope, I chose the new one which was three and a half hours north, in February, where I knew nobody, long before the internet was useful. Good choice!

I was accepted at the clinic and was really excited about learning from them. One of the doctors was well known for his ridiculous level of expertise, speed and accuracy for preg-checking cattle and I couldn't wait to pick his brain and find out his tricks. They had a small animal practice as well, but I made my intentions very clear at the interview that I was there for the livestock education. They were surprised but accommodating (most of the interest and focus in vet medicine is placed on small animal medicine). Great! Hmmm...now where am I going to live for a month? Small problem. I guess I was kind of hoping that the staff would know of a place, but no luck. The hotels in the area were astronomically priced, and any rentals wanted a minimum of 6 months' rent. Crap. Luckily after a lot of searching, I found out that one of the girls in my class knew of some guys that lived "kind of near there". (about a 40 min drive in good weather). Woohoo! I talked to them on the phone, agreed on a reasonable price and started packing. My parents were just thrilled with the idea of me moving in with 4 guys I didn't know, in a rundown old farmhouse in the middle of nowhere 4 hours away. Great idea! Luckily for all of us, the guys were perfect gentlemen who I rarely even saw due to all our conflicting schedules and I didn't even hear them much because I was living in the attic. Yep, the attic. They had said they had a small room for me which I had foolishly assumed was in the heated part of the house - silly me. They did provide me with a little space heater, but it was less than effective in the drafty old attic. I literally slept in pajama's, a jogging suit, my insulated coveralls for work, several pairs of socks a sleeping bag and sheets and blankets. It was terrible. Nowadays, I would have laughed at the conditions, walked downstairs and taken over a couch or even a spot on the floor, but back in my invincible days I just sucked it up because I didn't want to be a nuisance and I was tough. It was a LOOOOONG month.

I had a fantastic time at the clinic, the 2 large animal guys were awesome and taught me a ton of stuff and took me all over the place. The resident tech (literally - she lived above the clinic) was this super friendly, tiny little lady who had a ton of bulldogs that filled her apartment with snores and snorts. I didn't have much to do with the rest of the staff, but I did get to work with the small animal vet once on a very important case.......the other doctor!

The senior vet had taken me out to do a routine herd health call and things were sailing along well. We were freezing our butts off but one of the plus's of working with cattle is their body heat and their wonderfully warm armpits. Any time your hands need some warming up, just stick them in and you are good to go in minutes (plus, cows don't seem to mind as much as horses - wimps) Anyways, we were almost done and the farmer asked the vet to remove a couple extra teats from some heifers - no problem (sometimes cows grow extra teats on their udder which need to be removed before they start producing milk which is a quick, minor procedure). The vet finished the first heifer who never even stopped eating and then moved onto the second. This one was a bit more concerned with him poking around down there and chose to jump like a kangaroo at precisely the wrong moment. He proceeded to slip and damn near chop off the end of his index finger! I thought I had a potty mouth, but this man gave new meaning to the word. Once he ran out of words, he looked at me and said, "Get me to the clinic. NOW!"

I was a bit shell-shocked for a millisecond, then sprang into action. He was a big guy, so I was very thankful he could still walk. I pushed a path through the heifers and got all the gates for him. We made it to the truck and he collapsed into the passenger seat, with the colour rapidly draining from his face and the blood rapidly draining from his finger. Luckily, I knew where he kept some bandaging supplies and I tossed them at him while I dove in the driver's seat and took off. I had never driven a great big dually before, but thankfully it was an automatic - he never would have made it if it were a standard! It was snowing, and I had very little idea where I was going but he was with it enough to direct me to the main road where I could take over. I jumped on the CB and told the clinic what had happened. They wanted him to go to the hospital, but he wanted the small animal vet to stitch him up. He didn't want to sit in emerge all day and he trusted her a lot more than a stranger. By the time we got back the other male vet was there and was able to help the injured man into the clinic and onto a chair. The female vet started cleaning the wound and told him several times to go to the damn hospital. He refused. She sighed and started drawing up the freezing. He stopped her and said, "Just do it." We all laughed, thinking he was crazy, this was a huge, deep laceration. He was not joking. After one last attempt to talk some sense into him, she gave up and started stitching. How he made it through that without passing out or punching her I will never know. He took one day off and then was back at. We've all had minor injuries or deep paper cuts on our fingers that throb for days, luckily it was not his working hand, but I can't imagine the pain he must have been in. Maybe that's part of the reason I didn't complain about living in the freezing attic, I didn't want to look like a wimp in front of this guy!

Diane

I met my friend Diane in my junior year of college. We hit it off right away. In our class of 40, the majority of students were very eager to don scrubs and work in clinics with companion animals (dogs, cats, exotics), there was also a few die-hard horse people. Diane came from a dairy and farming background and I had experience in clinic and with horses but was looking to get into dairy, which is why I chose an agricultural college. We both ran with different circles, but always enjoyed each other's company and hung out regularly.

Diane is a one in a million woman. She is the most real, down to earth, straight forward, generous, wonderful person. The best part though, is that there's no bull shit and no drama.

We kept in contact after college but a few years after I moved out west and we kind of lost touch for a bit. When I moved back, close to our Alma Madre (see Mr. Samson story) I actually ended up living on the same road as her sister's family about 3 miles away. One day soon after I moved there, I was sitting outside, and a minivan went speeding down my dirt road (strange) slammed on the brakes and reversed (even stranger because we didn't get any traffic). I was a little concerned. That is, until she got far enough up my driveway that I could see her waving. We ran up to each other both talking at once and she put out her arms, dropped them and punched me in the shoulder! We both laughed because neither of us were huggers, but we were so excited to see each other.

Throughout the next decade or so as I moved around, I always made visiting her a priority. We could go long stretches without seeing each other and pick up right where we left off, relaxed, easy, fun. I also used to (and will continue to ....right Diane?) run my dogs on her farm too. She has hundreds of acres and a gator (4 wheeler) and a pond and bush and when my big boys needed to burn off some energy, it gives me an excuse to go and visit.

One of my dogs and I even rented a room off her and her family for a couple weeks while I was in the process of moving to a new house, but my job started before I had possession of the new place.

When I was hospitalized, Diane was like an angel (don't worry, I won't get too sappy Diane!). She visited me regularly and brightened my day every time. I still have no idea how she managed it because she has 4 kids, a farm and a house to run and a successful business with her husband. But come hell or high water that lovely lady made the hour long journey many times and I can't thank her enough - even though sometimes she brought her pain in the ass husband (just kidding Doug!) She kept me sane because she didn't treat me any different and neither did Doug. They still bugged me, teased me and gave me a hard time and made me feel like, well, me! One time she even brought another friend of ours, a huge bag of garlic and we sat and peeled garlic for her yearly pickle making! Talk about multitasking. Most people would have said they were too busy, but not her, she just made me work. That was definitely one of the highlights of my incarceration.

She also gave me a special gift. You see, we were 99% sure that I was going to have a C-section and I had been harassing the staff continually to allow me to watch the birth. I was vehemently told no over and over again. I was adamant that I watched. Everything about this pregnancy had been taken out of my control and I'll be damned if I was going to let anyone steamroll me on this one. I tried everything, asking for a mirror, asking for the surgical drape not to be placed as a barricade under my chin - still no.

I was devastated. There was going to be a room full of people seeing my baby be born - but not me. Not gunna happen guys. I dug my feet in even harder and went to the higher ups. I finally convinced my doctor to allow me to have a video camera in the room - but she only agreed under the condition that it was her doing the surgery. If I had to deliver with another doctor, it was up to them. Finally! Some headway. Now I had 2 problems; first, no one knew when I was delivering and second, I didn't have a camera.

In walk Diane and Doug one night on their way to dinner and a movie. They brought me junk food (yum!) and a small pink bag. I devoured the fast food but opted to wait on the gift. I knew all too well their twisted sense of humor and had already received a gag bra, etc. They left for their movie. I opened the bag and found a compact video camera. Holy shit. I freaked out and called and left messages on their phone thanking them profusely. I was stunned. And now I was even more determined to make this happen.

When delivery day finally came, it was good news and bad news. Unfortunately, my doctor was not there but my dream team of nurses was. One of them even switched operating rooms to be with me. They all knew how desperately I wanted this once in a life time moment filmed and they agreed to bring the camera in. They got a med student to film and when the attending doctor was done surgery, he insisted on seeing it first, but then ok'd them to give it to me. HALLEHLUIAH! Thanks to Diane and Doug and some persuasive amazing nurses and I was able to see my son being born.

You'd think that would be enough good deeds eh? Nope. Not for Diane and Doug. When my relationship was falling apart with my son's father, they allowed me to live in their basement part time with my infant son. And once their rental apartment on the farm property came available, they let us move in. Then became my personal therapists. Diane for all the emotional, worrisome, panicked, new mom stuff and Doug for the have a beer and f**k it stuff! They provided me, my son, my Boz and my horse with a safe place to live and go through the tumultuous next few years.

There are definitely no words guys to express my gratitude and show my appreciation but there sure is a special place in heaven waiting for you both. THANK YOU.

Friends, Neighbours and Surprises

Right after college I moved into a farm house with my boyfriend and 2 of his buddies (it seemed like a good idea at the time...) The next farm to the east was home to 3 more young guys that worked with my boyfriend. We all had lots of fun and I stayed there for about 2 years. During that time there were lots of stories to tell but there are 3 that stand out in my memory.

1.   I was working at a dairy barn milking cattle, delivering calves and doing the grunt work for feed research trials (blood samples, milk data). Needless to say, the hours were insane, and the work was hard. We worked 10 days on and 4 days off, 12-14 hours a day. I loved the cows and had an awesome group of guys to work with, even though they teased me mercilessly. Obviously, the first day off every two weeks was a blissful time for me that first and foremost included sleeping in past 4:30 am. The roommates were all painfully aware that waking me up on that first day was going to have severe consequences. For the most part the fear of being physically assaulted by a 5'2" sleep deprived female with a 2x4 kept them in line.

However, one morning I got a tentative tap on the door which I ignored. Then a louder one which brought violent images into my mind, but I still ignored. Then a few distant cries of "Holy shit!". Then all 3 of them were in my room all talking at once. I sat up in bed cursing them all with a string of expletives nasty enough for a stunned moment of silence. Finally, one of them said, "But we don't know what to do! There's a horse looking in the front window!" With one more mumbled threat I got out of bed, stumbled to the living room and sure as shit, there he was! We had been visited by large male peacock several times from a neighbouring petting zoo who used to fight his reflection in our big living room window and scare the crap out of us, but never a horse.

So, as they all stood there with their mouths open, I pulled on my boots and sunglasses, went out to my car and got a halter and lead rope (luckily, I kept my own horses tack in my car). I walked up to the trespasser and he was a perfect gentleman. I yelled back at the guys to get to work trying to find the owner and I set off on an hour long walk to the closest farm that had horses. Keep in mind that I set off in pyjama's, rubber boots and Medusa bed head down a fairly busy 2 lane highway. I didn't even know if the horse was theirs, but he was a fat little bugger, so I didn't figure he'd strayed too far. I was so pissed off at getting woken up that I literally walked right up their driveway, opened the nearest paddock, led him in, took my tack and walked all the way back home without even going to the house to talk to them!! Once back in bed, I realized I should have said something but all I could think about was sleeping. Can you imagine their surprise when they realized they had an extra horse??

P.S. Thanks for waiting around to give me a ride back arse-holes!!

2.   In the height of our drinking/partying days at this house, our neighbours and us went to a big party together. We were all a mess. Half way through the night, one of the neighbour's ex-girlfriends showed up. Weeeee. Drama. Anyways, we pretty much ignored them while at the party and luckily, she went back to their place after. Our house all dropped into our beds and fell asleep. Within an hour we were woken up by yelling and fighting in our driveway. Then by our door slamming ....brief pause....glass breaking..........girl crying! My ex got up and went to see what was going on. He came back white as a ghost, stammering something like "blood everywhere, Tyler, can't look, gunna barf!" So, I got up and as I neared the back door the girl's cries turned into screams. I was very surprised to see that my ex hadn't exaggerated (he was very squeamish and could pass out from a paper cut). There was blood EVERYWHERE and lots of broken glass.

Not knowing what the hell had happened I just put on my drill sergeant hat and started yelling orders. First, get her outside and quiet. Second, get me clean towels and duct tape (hey, you gotta use what you have). Third, someone start a vehicle. The next 15 minutes were nuts, but the guys got the drama queen settled, I got Tyler's arm bandaged and we (Tyler, his ex, Kyle and I) loaded in the car and started the 30 plus minute drive to the nearest hospital. We were all surprisingly sober by the time we got there and then had to wait about 2 hours for him to be seen. He ended up getting dozens of stitches to his fingers and forearm.

On the ride back home, we got a rundown of what happened. Apparently, drama girl had threatened him that if he didn't get back together with her, she'd run over to our house claiming he'd beat her up. (FYI, he never laid a hand on her and she admitted to us in the car it was all BS, but never did apologize to him). Anyways, he followed her across the corn field, but she was faster and got in our house and locked him out (we started locking our doors the very next night to keep out crazy ladies!). He decided to open the window with his fist in order to reach the deadbolt. His arm got stuck in the glass. He proceeded to pull it back out. Eeeeewww.

In summary: Tyler and drama girl never saw each other again. He healed up nicely. I got home exhausted and hung over and had to clean up broken glass and what seemed like several bucketfuls of now congealed, clotted, sticky blood off our door, walls and stairs. Most people only have wildlife to be concerned about when they live out in the country, but we learned that drunken, dramatic princesses are far more dangerous and messy!

3.   While living at the same house, our college had an alumni pub that we were very excited to go to. We had only been out a couple years, so we were really eager to see everyone and catch up (no Facebook back then)

One of my closest friends was coming with her new boyfriend and since I lived about 15 minutes from the campus, they were going to crash with us. The pub was great. You can't go wrong with college friends and booze. Two thumbs up! The ride home was uneventful and sleeping arrangements were easy. Kyle and I in my room, roommate #1 in his room, Diane and Doug in roommate #2's room on the extra bed since he was working nights.

The next morning, we go out to find roommate #2 sleeping on the couch. He looks up sleepily and says, "I never saw who the hell's in the other bed in my room, but I know one of their names is "Oh Doug!" We collapsed on the floor laughing! Poor guy got off work early, came home, climbed into his bed in the dark and was more than a little surprised to be woken up to 2 strangers getting it on (rather loudly no less) Diane and Doug were 10 shades of red when they came out and our abuse started!

This is one of my favorites. It's short and sweet (and sassy) and to this day I can still get a rise out of her when I bring it up and retell it to someone new...........I think she'll be very happy to know it's now in a book!

Out West

Shortly after college, my friend Katrina and I decided to pack up and move out to B.C. We were young and dumb and full of dreams. We literally opened a map, closed our eyes and pointed - then moved there! We both split with boyfriends to make the move. Hers was not a big loss but mine - well, I didn't appreciate him enough when I had him and didn't realize what a keeper he was until it was too late.

Anyways, we packed our cars, got our "Trip Tix" from CAA (long before the days of GPS), and headed out....IN JANUARY. (I mentioned being young and dumb right?) Seemed logical at the time to drive across the country in winter, to a place we'd never been, to live in some guys basement granny flat we'd never met. We encountered snowstorms, very scary rest stops, getting lost and some kick-in-the-teeth doses of WTF have we gotten ourselves into.

One day when we were heading into Chicago, I steeled myself for the upcoming few hours (I hate driving in big cities and my friend could get lost in a parking lot) I was comforted by my dear fathers' reassurance that Chicago was no worse than Toronto, which I also hate driving in. I repeated his words over and over as my stress controlling mantra. Let me be the first to tell you all that Chicago is WAY fricking worse than Toronto and that my father is a big fat liar! Getting through the city was bad enough, but once you get on the expressway, all hell breaks loose. There's approximately 5000 lanes of traffic all going 200km/hr, then slamming on their brakes at toll booths every flipping 2 km. Oh ya, you can see the exit signs as they fly by you with no warning 12 lanes away but good luck getting over to them to get off. That is the first and only time in my life I have ever wanted to curl up in the fetal position and cry while driving.

We made it through (I don't know how) and got to a hotel. I walked in the room, called my dad immediately (shoes still on) and tore him a new hind end. He took it all very well - laughing hysterically and said, "if I told you how bad it was you never would have done it!" Arrrrggghhh! What kind of twisted ass logic is that?? That is the first time I screamed at him, swore directly at him and hung up on him. Once we recovered and were on our way the next day, the rest of the drive was uneventful.

We arrived in the teeny town of Peachland (the destination scientifically chosen by blind pointing) and started up the mountain. Up, up, up, up. We had never seen anything like it. When we finally arrived, we were stunned at the property. It was gorgeous. The house was beautiful and 1/2 built into the mountain. The property was several horse pastures that ended at a sheer drop off of a rocky cliff. Amazing. The landlord wasn't there yet but had told us to go on in to the basement apartment when we got there. We unpacked a few necessities and waited.

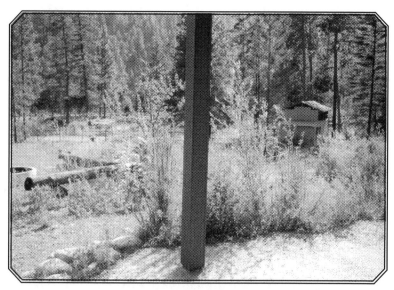

The view from our backdoor.

At some point he got home, came down and sat on the floor - back against the wall, knees up and proceeded to creep us out as his junk pushed through the hole in the crotch of his pants. We suddenly felt every single kilometer between us and home. Luckily for us, he turned out to be a harmless creep who ended up being quite popular with the local ladies........eeeeeewww. How do I know this you ask? Well, not only did he have and outdoor hot tub that shared a wall with my bedroom, but he also had his bedroom directly over top of mine. Eeeeewww. I got the stomach-turning pleasure of hearing many of his dates. I tried earplugs, pillow over my head, playing music - nothing could drown it out. The ickyness of what was happening permeated all of my barriers. The worst part is that I knew the dude's playbook - he was so predictable. To this day, I still shudder with repulsion when I hear Enya...........yep, that's right. The guy got his sexy on to a bunch of monks chanting!! Eeeewww.

While living out there I had three wildlife encounters that will stay with me for the rest of my life. The first one happened while I was taking my dog out for his last pee of the night. It wasn't just dark, it was black hole dark. There were no streetlights and our backdoor light had burnt out weeks prior. I didn't go more than 10 feet from the door when suddenly my body froze, my heart raced and all the hair on the back of my neck stood straight up. I pulled on my dogs' leash and spun to head back inside. I had no idea why I was freaking out, but the strength of that all-encompassing intuition was not to be ignored. As I spun, I saw eyeshine in the bush only 10-15 feet away that was about waist high. It may have only been a racoon in a tree, it may have been something far more dangerous – I don't know but I made it back in the house without my feet ever touching the ground! We did have mountain lions in the area and one of our neighbours had lost their puppy to a violent attack about a month prior complete with a blood trail and mountain lion tracks in the snow. The thing that bothered me the most was that my dog didn't react at all. I mean, he wasn't the smartest pooch I've ever had but you'd think some innate knowledge would have alerted him to a huge predator stalking his mom?? Guess not.

The other encounter happened while I was walking the same dog (in the daytime) down around the horse pastures in the fall. We were headed through some pretty tall grass and suddenly we came to a large clearing where all of the grass had been flattened in a circular pattern. Again, I froze and quickly took stock of the situation. Flattened grass, fresh blood stains, what's that over there....oh nothing, just a deer tail that had been ripped off and left bleeding on the ground. Holy shit! THIS time the dog was going nuts and I had to drag him all the way back to the house as I was sprinting for my life. Whatever animal was responsible for killing this deer was obviously large enough to take me out with zero problem, so I wasn't going to stick around. My only hope was that it was now so stuffed with deer that it didn't have the desire for a second course. Thankfully my dog and I both made it home, out of breath but alive.

The last memorable moment happened on a day my roommate and I were both home and getting ready for work. We had the tunes blaring but I still heard something weird and ignored it several times before asking her if she heard it too. We shut off the music and listened again. The next screech made us both jump and we ran to the patio doors to see what was going on. The screeching was getting louder but we couldn't see anything, so we assumed some poor critter was getting attacked in the bush, felt bad for it but continued getting ready. My friend left for work first, but she didn't get far. Once out of the house and headed up the hill to her car she spotted the problem – an emu was in our round pen! Not something you see everyday. She ran back in and called the landlord while I ran down the hill and shut the gate to contain the stressed-out bird.

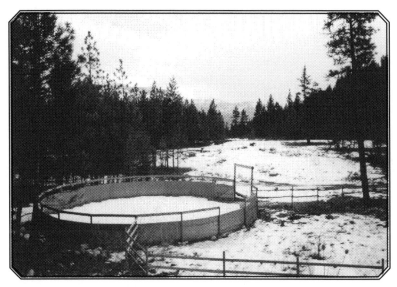

Scene of the crime.

Emus are not as big as ostriches, but they are definitely big enough to do some serious damage. Luckily, the round pen walls were tall enough to keep him inside. The landlord knew of an emu farm a few kilometers away and gave them a call. My friend went to work but I was lucky enough to be able to stick around for a while and watch 3 men try to load the emu into a horse trailer without being kicked. It was definitely entertaining and definitely memorable!

Eye

I have had the extreme displeasure of dealing with migraines since the age of 12. They are always very specific in their location (behind my left eye), so when I got some severe pain behind my right eye in June 2006 I was surprised. It wasn't exactly migraine pain, but it was intense and very localized, so I assumed it was just a strange version of one. I took my migraine meds, which didn't work. I took OTC meds, which didn't work. I endured a very long day at work.

The next morning, the pain was the same and I had lost some of the central part of my vision in my right eye. I was concerned but not panicked because over the years, I had had many vision issues accompanying the migraines. I did call the Dr while at work because it was proving to be a nuisance (hard to focus on a tiny ferret vein or look in a microscope, etc). The Dr said it was probably just a new issue surrounding the headaches and to take more meds and rest my eyes. So, I took the afternoon off work and did as I was told (rare!). By that evening, it had become much worse. Kind of like holding a black plate close to your face. I could see peripherally, but absolutely nothing straight ahead. So, off I go to emerge and saw the first 3 Dr's of my epic journey. They said to go home and come back in the morning when there was a more experienced Dr on duty. Fair enough.

The next morning, I woke up, yawned, stretched, hit snooze....then sudden, gut wrenching realization hits - I'm blind in my right eye! WTF?! I jumped out of bed, ran to the bathroom at mach 9. Yep. Sure as shit. BLIND. Luckily at the time, my ex was there and was able to drive me to the hospital (the only useful thing he proved capable of). I saw several more Dr's. They were stumped but at least were able to refer me on to one who was supposed to be the best. I have LOTS of other words for this man, but "the best" is certainly NOT on my list. He and his herd of underlings (various degrees of doctor-iness) checked me out for quite a while. He then proceeded to talk about me and my case to them, completely ignoring me (we were all in a teeny tiny room together).

Every time I interjected when he had a fact wrong or I had a question, I was either ignored with a rude look or shushed like a noisy kid in a movie theatre. He preceded to tell them that he thought I had a brain tumor. A fucking brain tumor. With the coldness and aloofness of someone talking about toe nail clippings. At this point, I lost it. I jumped up from the chair and yelled. He turned on me like a snake who'd had his tail stepped on.

"What do I do??", I begged.

"Get an MRI."

"OK and what if that doesn't show anything?", relaxing a bit since he finally spoke to me.

"Sigh....be thankful it's not a brain tumor." And with that he walked out of the room. His main minion didn't skip a beat, "We'll call you with your MRI appointment." and she followed Dr A-hole out.

I was left sitting in the exam room terrified, alone and shaking. When I came out, my ex (who by the way had the emotional maturity of a banana) looked like a deer in the headlights. We made it to his car, then I blurted out "brain tumor" and completely broke down.

After a week of waiting for a call, I called Dr. A-hole's office and was given the red tape run around. I'm usually pretty controlled and professional but that day I let loose with both barrels. "Perhaps it's not clear on your paperwork, but I'm fucking BLIND! I know there's a long wait for MRI's, but I also know there's emergency slots and I'm pretty fucking sure that if one of your daughters were going through this, she'd already have an appointment! I've been off work and stressed out of my mind because you asshole's told me I have a brain tumor. You think maybe we could figure this shit out a little quicker???!!!" I was out of breath and crying when I stopped my rant. The receptionist put me on hold and when she came back, I had an appointment booked 2 days later. Not proud of my behaviour but it was effective.

During this torturous month of my life, I ended up seeing 24 different doctors in 21 days - none of which did anything helpful until #24. Dr. N was a neurologist and an ophthalmologist. He was very grandfatherly, probably in his late 60's, early 70's with more credentials on his wall then I'd ever seen. He was wonderful. He had the answers, he had a bedside manner and he had bad news. he said I had optic neuritis. Basically, the nerves from the back of my eye to my brain got pinched by swelling and were now dead. The bad news was that if any of the previous 23 Dr's had given me a simple, basic course of steroids to bring down the swelling early on, I probably would have regained some, if not all of my sight. He said at this point it was pretty much useless to do but worth a try (21 days too late). He said it would be like tying an elastic band around the tip of your finger and leaving it there a month, then loosening it a bit - the damage had already been done. Fuck me sideways.

So, he issued the requisition for the steroid injections and sent me down to the lab asap for my first one. Now this wasn't a simple poke in the ass, it ended up being a slow IV drip. The nurse had to place a long-term catheter, so I could continue getting these IV's over the next 5 days. Once the drip started, it was annoying at best. It felt cold going in (even though the bag had been warmed), it made me itchy all over and quite strung out and agitated (like I drank 10 coffees). Finding it nearly impossible to sit still, I made it through with the knowledge that the next 5 days would be easier because I was getting a nurse to come do home visits since I lived in the country. Better, right? Come on now. You know better by now!

The first visits were uneventful, but the last was a joke. I was dreading sitting through it again, but I was happy that at least I'd get this friggin thing out of my arm today. The nurse came in all frazzled and late, then had to run back to her car several times for supplies. She talked a mile a minute and her hands shook. Not instilling a lot of confidence in me. She looked confused and fumbled with the equipment. I am not a human nurse, nor will I ever pretend to be one, but I am an RVT and I have placed thousands of catheters and maintained thousands of IV bags and lines in critters of varying sizes, species and locations. I tried not to overstep or insult but offered my 2 cents worth several times. It was my body after all and if there's anything I've learned from my medical journey, it's that you have to speak up and stand up for your own health.

She seemed ok and even appreciative of what I was saying. At one point I reached up and shut off the drip line. She looked stunned and I pointed out that more than half the line was full of air! She looked panicked, so I asked for a needle to insert in the extra port to vent the air. She looked confused, then checked her supplies. Nope. You came to do an IV procedure without friggin' needles??? Deep breath. Lucky for us, I kept a few small-bore sterile needles for splinter removal, so we got those and started trucking. She also needed one to draw up and inject the steroid into the bag. Guess she wasn't a Girl Scout.

One thing about steroids is that they have to be given slowly. I knew this from my veterinary training but also because all the previous, competent nurses had taken between 45-60 minutes to run the whole bag into me. This woman was doing her best Mario Andretti impersonation and trying to run it in as fast as possible. I talked to her several times, but she kept saying "it's fine, it's fine" (interesting side note, that is my most hated, most reactive phrase. I find it incredibly dismissive and condescending). Eventually, I turned it down myself while she was flustering about. Not an enjoyable day. When it was finally done, I don't know who was more relieved - her or me.

She disconnected me and instructed me to go back to the hospital to have the catheter removed. WTF??

"You're a nurse, can't you do it?"

"No, you have to go back."

"I'll do it."

Gasp! "No!"

"Ok, I'll go back in."

She wasn't out of my darn driveway and I had that damn catheter and the 8 miles of tape off. The bitch of it was that even after all that, the friggin' steroids didn't do anything and I'm still blind in my right eye to this day. Grrrr.

28

After my eye issues, the doctors thought I had Multiple Sclerosis. Shit. So, I went through several MRI's and a multitude of testing and countless new doctors. The final conclusion was that I did indeed have MS. A devastating blow to say the least. However, I never believed it. I can't explain why. I knew there was lots of evidence and the doctor and specialist were making their best educated guess but, in my gut, I just didn't believe it. Not because I was in denial or delusional, it just didn't sit right with me. (FYI MS is not a black and white diagnosis. It is a huge grey area).

I was lucky enough to have parents who could afford to take me to the Cleveland Clinic in the states for a 2nd (thirteenth) opinion. We were blown away by the experience. Top notch is the best phrase I can come up with. The hospitality, the care, the staff, the doctors, the lack of wait times. Long story short, their MS specialist quickly discovered that I did not have MS but instead had lupus. Shit again. Not the word I wanted to hear, but definitely the lesser of the 2 evils. I came back north armed with his report and ended up being referred to hands-down one of the best doctors I have ever had the privilege of knowing. Dr. T. was like a gift from above. He's compassionate, approachable, understanding and actually has a sense of humor. After a thorough intake exam and history, he gave me a 5-page requisition form to take to the lab. I've had a lot of tests done in my life, so I wasn't too shocked considering the immensity of the situation. My mom had driven me to the appointment that day because I was still adjusting to the whole one eye thing. She sat in the small waiting room while I went in. The lab tech took the papers and started reading. She looked up at me several times with a strange look in her eyes. Now I was getting concerned. She then excused herself and had a whisper conversation with another lab tech. This process was repeated again. Yep. Worried. They came back over.

"Your doctor has ordered A LOT of tests. Do you want to lay down while we do this?"

As I said, I'm no stranger to getting poked and prodded so I said no, I'd stay in the chair. They looked doubtful but proceeded getting their gear ready as my feeling of apprehension grew with each passing second. You know those tackle boxes they carry around the hospital full of supplies? They brought 2 over beside me. Then they arranged themselves in an assembly line - no joke. Tech #1 was the poker, using a large bore butterfly catheter. Tech#2 was the hand off for the full blood vials and the labeller. Tech #3 was the paperwork checker and packager of the samples. Tech #4 was handling the computer work. They were an amazing, well oiled machine. (Thank heavens!) After what seemed like an eternity and several more concerned inquiries into if I'd like to lay down, they finished. As I was putting pressure on the needle site and feeling like Count Dracula had just had his way with me, Tech #1 shook her head and said,

"Well that was a first! I've never pulled that much from someone at one sitting!"

"More than I've ever sat for, that's for sure!" I echoed.

"Honey, we just pulled twenty-eight 10ml vials from you!"

They made me sit there for about 10 minutes and drink juice before I could leave. I felt ok, so I said my thanks to them and headed out. My mother's eyes were pretty wide as she had heard the whole thing out in the waiting room!

Thanks to Dr. T's thoroughness, we had a diagnosis confirmed, and could get started on a battle plan. Not great news to have lupus but news that my body didn't reject with the vehemence it did with the MS diagnosis. I was happy to kiss MS goodbye (for now......duh, duh, duh....foreshadowing!) and start being able to focus on and fix my current situation.

Lupus, aka the disease of 1000 faces (because the symptoms are so varied) ended up being a tricky pain in the ass too, but I'm still here and not in a wheelchair, so let's get ready for round 592!

Arsenic

During the many years of strange symptoms, fear and misdiagnosis I experienced a myriad of emotions - mostly negative. My strictly science-based, analytical mind was forced into widening a teeny bit to explore other health care options. I started small and still have lots of scepticism and difficulty accepting some of the more "woo woo" concepts. My logic though has always been governed by cold, hard facts and proof. My life has centred around animals, so I started out with things that I had seen work for them since they don't know how to lie, and they aren't fooled by placebo affects. The first step was chiropractic care. I had seen chiropractic work for both horses and dogs. I had seen difficult to handle animals (probably due to pain) become as malleable as Play-doh after only a few minutes of treatment, so that's where I started. I found a husband and wife team of doctors who ran a very laid-back practice. They were great, their work was great and the environment there was wonderful. After a short while, I was seeing real tangible benefits with my decreasing amounts of daily pain, and it spurred me on to seek out some more alternative health care. I even invested in a magnetic mattress pad which was supposed to help alleviate pain. The day I put it on my bed I discovered that it did other things too – like attract all of my critters! I came into my room and found 2 large dogs and 2 cats peacefully laying together directly on top of the new pad (even though they were not allowed on my bed!). I quickly realized that there must be something to alternative health care stuff.

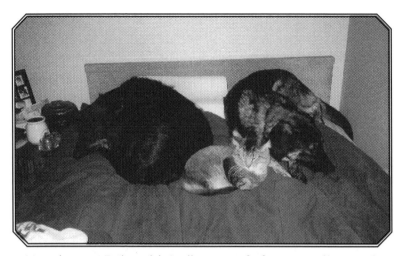

My other cat Evil couldn't allow proof of getting along with the others, so she took off when I grabbed the camera.

Next came a fantastic naturopath who I met through Annabel. She was awesome and was excellent at dialing back the "woo woo" to an acceptable level for me while still exploring areas ignored by western medicine or using different tactics to work on already diagnosed issues. She was wildly intelligent and compassionate, and I quite enjoyed her sleuthing ability and methods. One of her biggest accomplishments with me was during our time of trying to figure out the autoimmune tornado swirling around me and all the weird stuff happening to me. She had a light bulb moment one day and quite literally jumped out of her chair. "Arsenic!" she yelled. Turns out arsenic poisoning can mimic a lot of the symptoms I had, and she immediately got excited and started a rapid-fire barrage of strange questions. Because of my history of growing up in the chemical valley, some questionable lifestyle choices, my work environments, exposure to years of radiation, chemicals and medications, old barns, well water, etc. etc. etc. she said it all made perfect sense. So, we chopped off a hair sample and sent it away and when it came back, sure enough, my arsenic levels were sky high!

Now there were 2 burning questions: 1. Where did I get it (and how do I stop getting it)? 2. How do I get rid of it? The first things we did were to check my well water (which did have arsenic "above acceptable levels") and draw blood to double check the hair sample results (which was also "above acceptable levels"). Interesting. Apparently, there's not a lot that can be done to extract arsenic from your body, but she gave me several treatments and remedies to help my body break it down and release it. It definitely was a strange diagnosis but a whole lot better than the alternative. It also empowered me and gave me some options and dare I say hope. An interesting side note is that in my OAC/grade 13 Writing class, I had written a short story on a woman who is being slowly poisoned WITH ARSENIC by her a-hole boyfriend! This was long before CSI and that movie the sixth sense! Co-incidence??

From there, I saw an iridologist who freaked me out with her accuracy but stumped both of us because everything she read was flipped (she'd say that my left shoulder was full of trauma, but it was my right). Not surprising that my body didn't read the rule book on that one.

Next, after I lost my sight, I saw an acupuncturist (which I had also seen work wonders in dogs, horses and cattle). My experience there was not so good. It's not the needles, I have lots of voluntary tattoos. It was the intensity, the language barrier, the complete lack of bedside manner that came with a very large dose of guilt and accusation. The doctor made you feel very judged and responsible for everything going on and was very rough and robotic. Not a great personality for someone jamming needles into you! He also lit a few on fire (controlled but still very ouch) and hooked some up to little alligator clips connected to electricity. I gave it a fair shake, but this was definitely not for me.

Lastly, the boss who fired me when I went blind in my right eye, because apparently, I was a "liability" now, gave me a parting gift of a book on alternative healing by Louise Hay which I ignored (but didn't throw out) for a long time but eventually read. That book opened up a whole new world for me, even though I tread into it like a timid little mouse finding her way through a gymnasium full of a million mouse traps. After reading that book, I read many more Hay House authors including Wayne Dyer, Nick Ortner, Mike Dooley, Iyanla Vanzant and more. Quite frankly my mind was blown.

In the end, it was all a very interesting journey that I definitely wouldn't have had if not for my health issues. I'm still blind in my right eye. I still have lupus. I still have a grey-area surrounding a fluctuating diagnosis of MS. But thanks to people willing to try new things and help out and have a different view (I'm really trying hard not to say "think outside the box"), I have been able to look at my stuff a little differently and with a lot more understanding, curiosity and hope.

Car Accident

One classic southwestern Ontario winter's day, I made the poor choice to travel on a two-lane highway that was known to be treacherous. I was actually going to a friend's house about an hour away to get her cat who I was re-homing for her. I knew it would be a crappy drive, but I had an awesome little jeep, huge snow tires, 4-wheel drive and a cautious driving record. As I slowly manoeuvred along, I came to a clearing where the road was finally free of copious amounts of the white stuff, so I breathed a small sigh of relief for a minute. That's when I hit the black ice. It all happened in slow motion.

My car spun around, and I kept moving in the original direction - so essentially, I was driving backwards in the opposite lane (thankfully no one was coming) then I hit more ice and proceeded to roll down the steep ditch. I rolled one full turn and then 1/2 more so I ended up on my roof. I was hanging upside down by my seatbelt, dazed. As I hung there, the only thing I could think of was that I had to get down. In my brain, which was not thinking logically at the time, it seemed like a good idea to undo my seatbelt. CRASH! I landed on the roof of my car with a thud. Perhaps I should have thought that one through a little more. I injured myself more from that than I had in the accident! The car landed in a huge pile of snow which cushioned my landing but also blocked all the doors. I was stuck. My logical brain was making a come-back and I started figuring out what to do. Coincidentally, my roommates cell phone was sitting in clear view (she had lost it a few days prior and the collision must have shaken it free from its hiding spot). I grabbed it and called her. There was not much battery life left, but I was able to fill her in and she hung up to call the cops.

While I waited there for what seemed like forever, I had noticed that my laundry basket full of dirty laundry had rolled and displaced my stuff all over the place. I was mortified and started crawling around the roof retrieving everything I could find. In hindsight, caring about the cops seeing my underwear certainly doesn't seem as important as my injuries but at the time it mattered. By the time I heard a vehicle, I was very sore and very cold. As I tried to see who was coming and realized it was a snow plow, I was relieved and scared at the same time. What if he slipped in and squashed me?! Luckily, he was able to stop, and he came down and started digging me out. I had never been so happy to see a complete stranger. He helped open the door and pull me out. Then he helped me climb the steep, snowy embankment and put me in his deliciously warm truck. He called his dispatch and told them what was happening. As I sat in the truck, I noticed a huge electrical transformer that my car had missed by only a few feet. I swallowed hard. My accident narrowly missed being a whole lot worse. A few minutes later the cops came, I thanked the driver profusely and transferred myself into the cop car (which was also nice and toasty). The officers were wonderful and as we sat there filling out paperwork and waiting for the tow truck, we watched in silence as another car hit the same patch of black ice as me and headed straight for us! I kid you not, the woman went into the ditch four feet in front of the cruiser. As she landed down in the ditch, we all let out a collective sigh of relief that she didn't hit us or my car which was not far away and would have made for a much tougher landing for her. All I could say was, "Yep, that's pretty much how it happened!". The cops jumped out to help her and told me to stay put. Several minutes later she came to join me in the back of the cruiser. We were both banged up and shook up but luckily no serious injuries.

After a week of dealing with insurance (fun) and tending to my boo-boo's and mooching rides to work life got back to normal. I did make sure I put an ad in the paper thanking the generous snow plow driver because I never got his name or company info and I wanted to make sure I tried my best to thank him. He definitely went above and beyond, and I sincerely hope he was able to read it. Young girls might dream of being rescued by a knight on a white horse, but my real-life hero was a sweet old man in a huge plow truck!

*　　*　　*　　*　　*

The only other time I was in an accident was TOTALLY not my fault. I know lots of people say that but, my car was parked! I had stopped at a rural gas station to fill up where they still have full serve. I was sitting in my car paying the attendant through my window then KERBLAM! My head hit my steering wheel and the attendant had disappeared from my peripheral vision. After a few stunned seconds I heard a lot of yelling - which was directed at me. WTF?? This a-hole of a truck driver had leaped out of his big rig cab and was cursing and swearing and flailing his arms while quickly making his way over to me. I was confused and more than a little scared. As he continued his barrage of insults the gas attendant finally stepped in and stopped the guy by saying, "I was standing right here buddy and I saw everything!" The truck driver stumbled over his words for a minute then picked up where he left off. Then another man at a different pump came over and told him to cool his jets because he saw it too. He swore for several minutes more then finally exchanged information with me and took off. After thanking the men, I finally found out what happened. I was parked with the engine off and this truck driver flew in backwards to the pump, obviously didn't see me and rear ended me hard enough to move my parked car about 6 feet. He tried desperately to convince me it was my fault but finally realized it was a lost cause. In hindsight of course, I should have called the cops, but everything happened so stinkin' fast and he took off, so I called my dad and let him handle it with the trucking company. We've all heard more than enough about women drivers but women parkers??? Come on!!

Clinics

During my 20's, I worked at a conglomerate of 5 veterinary clinics which spanned a couple of local towns for 4 years. It was great because of my propensity to get so flippin' bored so quickly and I was able to head to a different clinic several times a week to keep life more interesting. We had a great crew. There were bosses/old people (looking back, not so old now!), and then the rest of us who were all in our 20's and 30's, all got along (for the most part) and all liked to party. It was a lot of fun and with that many people, there was always something going on. Two memorable stories stand out from my time there.

1.   While I was relatively new at one of the clinics, I noticed (too late) that all the other techs and support staff disappeared at the same time. As I looked around in wonder, one of my favorite vets came back to the treatment room and asked for my help. He handed me a tray of supplies and beckoned me to follow. As I glanced down at the tray, I realized why the other tech's bailed on me. It was full of semen collection equipment. Shit heads.

Now, let me clarify, vet clinics strive to uphold a very professional standard, but we are human. And I don't care how mature you THINK you are, when you see a grown man on his knees, whacking off a dog, it's friggin' funny! I mustered my courage and tried to think of ANYTHING else as I entered the room. Unluckily for me, the owners wanted to watch. The keep-a-straight-face ante was just upped substantially.

The dog was a large, old, arthritic German Shepherd who apparently had amazing bloodlines but was unable to mount the female anymore, so that's where we stepped in. One owner held the dog's leash, the other paraded the female in heat in front of him. My job was to keep the DVM supplied with the necessities and to take the sample once collected to our lab. Here we go. The old dog was quick to react to the female and the Dr got to work (you're picturing it now aren't' you?). I stared holes in the floor, literally biting my cheek, hoping the pain would avert any laughter. The old dog had a difficultly after a few minutes and the Dr had to increase his efforts to compensate for the dogs decrease in movement. Help me Jesus. Then the grunting started. The dog from exhaustion, the Dr from exertion. In a last-ditch effort to stop a river of laughter from busting through the wobbly mental dam I had constructed, I bent my leg the wrong way and sat on it hard - success! That hurt! And then, success! The old fella burst through his own dam!

I quickly gathered the sample from the Dr and hurried back to the lab where I was met by the rotten S.O.B.'s that threw me under the bus. We all burst out laughing while I swore a blue streak and physically harmed a couple of them. We pulled it together by the time the Dr came back. We analyzed the sample (all good) and then the Dr and I headed back in to deal with the female. This would be a cake walk compared to the first half.... right?

We positioned her up on an exam table, owner at her head, my shoulder under her belly to keep her standing, one hand holding her tail out of the way, the other free to help the vet. Everything was going smoothly as he inserted the catheter and attached the syringe full of liquid gold. Things changed abruptly when he started to inject. As the jet of still warm semen shot out and hit me in the forehead, we all realized he had not tightened the syringe enough. Seriously. I wish I were joking. I froze in stunned, repulsed silence. The owner gutted himself with laughter, the Dr's mouth dropped open in surprise and then without missing a beat, he grabbed a new syringe and tried to suction some of it off my face as it was running down the side of my nose. Luckily, he still had more than enough left in the original syringe and we were able to finish the artificial insemination successfully.

As soon as we were done, I flew into the bathroom and began washing my face about 1000 times. When I emerged, I was met by applause and a chorus of laughter. I was the brunt of some pretty sick jokes for months.

I've always been a supporter of adopting from shelters instead of breeding.........now, even more so!!

*　　*　　*　　*　　*

2.   I was working with a young vet who I got along with well (he was actually dating a friend of mine). We were in surgery working on a cat, removing a piece of bowel. We worked well together, and everything was going along great (1st warning sign of impending doom).

Once he entered the abdomen and found the piece that needed to come out (about 4") I scrubbed in and held the bowel an inch away from the offending tissue on either side, using my first and second fingers (like making pretend scissors). You just tried that didn't you? By using this grip, the healthy tissue wouldn't be damaged, and I could apply enough pressure to prevent the contents from leaking out. everything was still going well, except for some minor finger cramps. I was in the middle of telling him a story from my weekend when I was abruptly interrupted by searing pain, "So anyways, blah, blah, blah....holy hell! Ow! WTF!?". Yep. The Dr had sutured the end of my left index finger to the cat (you just can't make this shit up). Somehow, he had pushed the very sharp, curved suture needle through my finger and through the bowel before I reacted. Thankfully for the cat,

I had the wherewithal not to let go or else the bowel contents would have spilled into the cat and he probably would have died from sepsis. So, I just stood there swearing and yelling for another tech to scrub in. As someone finally heard me and rushed to scrub and glove the Dr was left with a new problem. The suture and suture needle are fused together and now since both had passed through my finger, he was going to have to start all over with a new set. After many LONG minutes, we were able to sever my ties to the cat, switch off with the other tech, the vet resumed surgery and I was finally able to attend to my throbbing finger.

Once the surgery was over and the cat was waking up the vet attempted to approach me several times. His outbursts of laughter prevented him from apologizing, but his brain wisely kept him back - just out of my strike range. Later that week he tried to make up for it by picking up the tab for a night of pool and whiskey and I let him off the hook. Looking back, I feel I was way too lenient!

The cat did beautifully and healed fast. He had no ill effects from his experience but every time he came in after that, the Dr stayed the hell away from me!

Food Poisoning

Thanks to my Brownie-ravaged guts, I have been extra sensitive to any kind of stomach bug or food poisoning for the rest of my life. There were a couple episodes that bear repeating.

A couple years after college I went to a reunion BBQ at a friend's farm. We were all having a great time catching up, partying and regaling each other with our new-found "grown up" stories. Everyone ate the same stuff - your classic BBQ fare - burgers, hotdogs, salads, beer, beer, beer. I felt pretty terrible the next morning but that kind of goes with the territory and I certainly don't expect any sympathy for self induced stupidity, so I sucked it up and got in the car for my long drive home. That 2 1/2 hours felt like about 24 hours. When I got home, I was at the point where you are bartering with the powers that be, "If you help me feel better, I WILL NEVER DRINK AGAIN.", "Please let me drink some water without barfing...PLEASE" and so on and so on. By that evening I was fairly sure I was either possessed or on my way out. I slept on the bathroom floor. I ended up missing a week and a half of work (the most I've ever missed in my entire working career!) and I couldn't even make it to the hospital because I could only go about 10 minutes without expelling the demons from my weak, sore, dehydrated body. During that time, I sustained myself on water and popsicles and I lost an incredible 14 pounds. After the first week, I was amazed that there was anything left to come out. I hadn't eaten in days, but both ends of my body were still productive. You know how they say that an average adult has like 5-7 pounds of undigested food stuck in their intestines? Not anymore. I'm pretty sure I pooped out my pancreas too! The worst part? NOT ONE of the other party-goers got sick....NOT ONE.

*   *   *   *   *

In my 20's my parents and I took a trip to Toronto to visit my brother and see one of his plays (the name of it escapes me now, you'll see why soon). We all went out to dinner and everything was lovely, the food was good, and we were having a good time. Side note, I even met my big brother's future wife that night even though he didn't believe me at the time when I pointed it out to him after she came up to the table to say hi!

After supper we went directly over to the theater, which was somewhere in the bowels of downtown T.O. - NOT my comfort zone, I'd rather be out in the sticks on horseback. Anyways, we got our seats and waited for the show to start. About 10 minutes into the performance I started to feel kind of gross. Nothing to be worried about yet, but just a bit queasy. The following several minutes deteriorated rapidly and I had the joy of experiencing nausea, sweating and the shakes. I soon realized that offending the actors and my brother by walking out was a WAY better alternative than my other option so as quickly and as quietly as possible I found my way out. It was an old, dark theater so this was tougher than you may think.

I finally got out into the lobby and searched frantically for a bathroom – ANY bathroom because the clock was ticking and at that moment I didn't care if I barfed in a urinal, a toilet or a garbage can! I couldn't find anything and was getting really worried because I knew there would be no avoiding the upcoming onslaught of my body forcefully purging whatever demon I had ingested. As the first little warning hiccup/burp/tiny heave hit me I gave up my search and ran for the doors. Luckily for all involved I made it outside. As the attack progressed, I made it further and further down the alley beside the theater, until I got too close to the garbage bins whose odor brought on more reaction from my taxed-out tummy. Exhausted and disgusting I leaned up on the wall trying to catch my breath.

That was when I saw them. A group of 7 young men boisterously talking loudly and roughhousing. I have no idea if they were part of a gang or not, but it was late, and they were walking down a nasty, dark alley. Funny thing was that I couldn't have cared less at that time! As they got closer and noticed me, everything about them changed. They stopped pushing and shoving each other, they quieted down into their "hey baby" voices and had a far more menacing air to them. Which I quickly shut down by launching into another round of projectile vomiting! They stopped dead in their tracks and as one unit moved to the other side of the alley without a word.

As I said, I have no idea who they were or what their plans were but who knew you could stop potential street violence with food poisoning?!

Annual

So, ladies, we can surely all commiserate with each other when thinking of or going through our yearly physical exam. The ultimate in humiliation, the most unflattering positions and fluorescent lights. Trying to desperately focus on counting the holes in the ceiling tiles while someone, inevitably with cold hands, is rooting around in our business. As if that wasn't bad enough, unfortunately, I can add yet another layer of misery to this experience.

My friends had finally convinced me to go on a vacation with them to Jamaica in my late 20's. I've always been frugal (my opinion) and a tightwad (their opinion) with money and I never like to spend it on frivolous stuff. But they swayed me over to the dark side.

While getting stuff ready for the trip, I realized I needed a refill on my birth control pills, so I called the doctor - who was away for 3 weeks! Shit. The nurse said I should go to a walk-in clinic, get the pap test and get a month's worth of pills, then I could see my doctor when she got back. I was very frustrated but stuck because I couldn't go off the pill especially in Jamaica because of my insane periods. So, I called around, found a clinic and headed over.

With sweaty palms, I waited for what seemed like an eternity and then the door opened, and the tiniest, nicest looking little Dr man came in with a nurse in tow. He smiled, patted my knee and gestured for me to "assume the position". Just as I laid my head back on the paper pillow case, I felt a punch in the crotch followed by searing heat in my nether-regions!! I sat bolt upright, while letting out a coyote wail only to find the Dr desperately fumbling with the stand-up exam light that he had accidently knocked over onto my lady bits! He said sorry about a million times and the poor young nurse was frozen with a perpetual deer in the headlight's expression. He finished fast and left the room. I got dressed and the nurse came back in with my prescription and a suggestion of a strategically placed ice pack for a couple days.

Upon calling my so-called friend to inform her of what happened, I was expecting some sympathy since it was her idea to go on this damn trip. I was sadly mistaken. To this day whenever either of us has to go for a physical she refers to it as going for a "crotch punch". Needless to say, Jamaica was awesome, except for the damn salt water........it stings!

Mr. Samson

Throughout my life I have lived in a lot of places (17 to be exact). One of the most memorable ones was just outside a little place called Ridgetown.

I had just moved back from out west and had less than 2 weeks to find a place to live because I had a job starting (going back to milking cows). I drove around for several days looking, I read all the local papers and talked to everyone I knew in the area (before the internet was what it is today young punks!). Finally, an old college teacher of mine pointed me towards this house but only with a very vague knowledge that it used to be a rental.

I drove out to this old farm house, knocked on the door, looked in the window and confirmed that it was empty. The closest neighbour was a couple miles away, so I decided to try my luck there. I banged on the door and waited ....for a while. Eventually this tiny elderly lady opened it and told me to come in. She seemed harmless enough, so I did. I tried dozens of times to ask her about the house, but she kept getting sidetracked telling me about the weather, recipes, her health concerns, etc. I'm not sure how much of that was boredom/loneliness vs. Alzheimer's/ senility but I persevered because I really needed a place! Finally, she understood what I was asking and said that of course she knew who owned the house, it was her son! Halleluiah! Now, to find out his number. She found his contact info with less trouble than I expected, handed it to me and I was off (much to her dismay). The sweet old lady wanted me to stay for lunch!

I called the man as soon as I got to my parent's place (no cell phone back then). To say I had to bite my tongue a few times while talking to him would be a huge understatement. It took me quite a while to convince him to let me come see the place because I was "just a girl", "had no husband" who "couldn't possibly handle living alone". Grrrrrr.

At this point, I had to call in the least likely of candidates to help me argue with a chauvinistic old man. My dad. A slightly less old, chauvinistic man. We headed out to the house the next day. The owner explained that it had been empty for a while because he didn't need the money and it wasn't worth the headache to rent it out. The house was in rough shape, not gross, just rough. Not one floor was level, if you dropped something you better be ready to move because you wouldn't know where it was going to roll to. It was small, it was old, and it needed a serious cleaning.

While the "men folk" were talking and I was internally cursing, a bat whooshed past us. The landlord casually reached under the sink, grabbed a small pot and lid and caught the little bugger without missing a beat! (a skill I would soon acquire....) Once the tour was done, he stood there, arms crossed and looked at me shaking his head and said, "I just don't think it's going to work. You're a GIRL. Who's going to do all the work around here without a man??". After swallowing a big lump of anger, I tried once again to explain that I in fact was not a useless waif incapable of caring for myself or starting a lawn mower. He ignored me and said (and I quote) "Sigh....I just don't want to get called over here every time a damn light bulb burns out."

At this point, luckily for me and for this sexist a-hole, my dad stifled his laughter and went to bat for me. I just stood there vibrating in stunned fuming silence. I was seriously considering what the criminal charges would be for kicking the shit out of a senior citizen. Now, I'm not a bra burning feminist, but I am a strong, independent, self sufficient, educated, hardworking PERSON and my tolerance was disappearing at an alarming rate.

Thankfully, we left the farm without incident and also the keys to my new place.

* * * * *

After the first week of living there I realized that I had to get a plan for cutting the grass. Not a big deal, right? Well, actually it is when the property was just over 3 acres and I had no lawn mower, and I worked very long hours for 10 days in a row. So, I would drive 1 hour each way, pick up my dad's push mower and a jerry can of gas and bust ass for the next 6 1/2 hours. I've never been in better shape! My 22-year-old body and my spitfire personality that wouldn't give this old fart the satisfaction of seeing me fail pulled me through! He drove by a few times that summer and saw me out there, would slow down and wave, but never said a word.

Even when my shower head and taps would randomly spit out big gobs of orange slime, I didn't call him. To this day, I still don't know what that crap was. I'd be showering, hear a weird noise, then feel something raw egg-like slide down my body....blech.

Even when 10 minutes after I'd go to bed at night my walls would literally come alive with the scurrying, squeaking and scratching of what I can only guess was thousands of rodents, I didn't call him. I had a removable chunk of flooring that would allow me to place traps in between the 2x4's. I could easily fill the 12 traps 2x day with 100% success. Eventually I stopped because there was no way I was even making a dent in their population, I felt bad nuking them and I was getting used to the "white noise" they provided.

I also became very proficient at catching bats with my little soup pot. Ridiculous thing was though, that I would let them go outside and I'm sure they'd fly right back up to wherever they were getting in! Probably thinking there was something very wrong with the crazy lady who kept catching them.

I ended up living there for over 2 years and I never called him to change a light bulb. :)

*   *   *   *   *

During my time renting from him, I had an insane experience one summer. I got home from work around supper time and my goofy dog was nowhere to be found. I was concerned, but not worried yet. I walked around the property calling and whistling, still no dog. I went in and got showered up, had a bite to eat and was surprised to find he had not returned yet. He never wandered for long and always came home by supper time. He wasn't much of a hunter, more of a sleeper/sun bather. I walked around again calling and whistling - nothing. So, I got my keys and started the car while calling him. What dog doesn't love a car ride? Success! I heard a far-off bark and then saw and heard the corn stalks rustling. I got up on my hood to get a better view since I'm vertically challenged and boy was I surprised.

There was 3 cop cars and I small black car in the middle of the next field over about a mile away and a very obvious trail being made from that direction to me. After a few minutes, Sherman (already named when I adopted him) came bouncing out of the corn. I was so relieved. I cleaned him up and brought him inside. He ate quickly then immediately plopped down and fell asleep. I wondered all evening what the hell was going on out in the field, but it was strictly curiosity, not fear since the cops were there and obviously had everything under control right? Not exactly.

The next day I tied Sherman up (much to his dismay) and headed out to work. I couldn't wait to ask my boss if he knew what was going on - he definitely had his finger on the pulse of the area. He knew everybody and was usually the first to know new information. He had heard about the cops in my area but didn't know why yet (keep in mind it was 4:45am). Well all that would change before I went for lunch.

Through his grapevine, he found out some disturbing news. Apparently, there was a gang fight in Toronto (about 4 hours away) and someone got killed. The killers threw the body in the trunk of their car and took off. The cops caught up with them and chased them along the highway. Bad guys panicked, took the off ramp 5 minutes from my place and went off road through the corn field in a teeny little civic-type car (good thinking guys). Obviously, they got stuck, the cops caught one of them, but the other guy got away, for the time being.

Here's where I freak out. I was so mad. So, there's a gang-banger who just killed someone running around in the corn behind my house and the cops decided there was no need to at least tell be to be on alert??? To lock my doors??? He's obviously dangerous, willing to kill, panicked and needing a place to hide and a car. Helllllooooo!! The cars were all parked between the 90-something year old lady and me a 20-something year old lady, both living alone in the middle of nowhere! Do you think maybe a heads up would have been a good idea boys??

Funny enough, that morning I had actually thought I would stop and bring them some coffee on the way home since they were still out in the field. Well not now! No coffee for you!

Halfway home that night, a realization hit me like a ton of bricks. Sherm had been over there. What if he'd seen, touched, sniffed the dead body?! What if the bad guy had hurt him? Why didn't the cops call me? (he had tags on) I was so fired up but then it dawned on me just how lucky I was that nothing had happened.

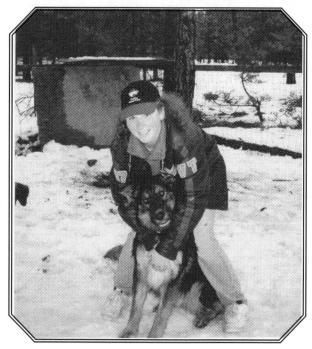

My "police dog" Sherman.

The cops stayed out there for 3 days processing evidence, I assume. I still think they should have warned me but once my initial rage simmered down, the only thing I could focus on was whether or not Sherman had licked the dead body. Eeeewwww!

The Night of 1000 Critters

I had a very memorable night about 10 years ago when I tried driving to my friend's house who lived 15 minutes away. We were both in the country and both used to the normal nocturnal wildlife we often encountered, but nothing could have prepared me for this.

As I headed out, I narrowly missed 3 squirrels who darted out on the road, one after the other only a few feet from my car. Since when do they travel in herds? My pulse quickened, I hit the brakes, no big deal, I drove on. Not far from there, I saw 4 different racoons (separately) in the span of about a mile - luckily all far enough away that I had plenty of time to stop. By this point, I was very curious about what game mother nature was playing with me. It was a chilly, early winter evening with a light dusting of snow, a crystal clear, black sky and zero wind. There was no reason for what was happening.

As I was contemplating the appearance of all these animals (and driving very slowly now) I got the shock of the night. A very large buck with a VERY large set of antlers was waiting in the middle of my lane as I came around a blind s-curve heading downhill! Both of our eyes got real big real fast, I slammed on the brakes and tried to avoid him. My car came to a stop sideways, straddling the yellow line and I was holding my breath waiting for the thud.........
which never came. As I finally let out the breath I'd been holding, I heard some scuttling and scratching and quickly saw that big rack rise up right beside my passenger window! I never hit him, but he must have fallen down trying to scoot away from the car. He righted himself, shook, looked right at me through the window, snorted and calmly walked off the road! I was sweating and shaking as I manoeuvred the car back into my lane. I looked back twice at the magnificent, albeit arrogant beast and he kept

staring at me as I drove away. Obviously frazzled, I thanked the powers that be that I had not been hurt nor hurt him and I drove on at about 10km/hr.

From that point, I encountered a bunch of racoons feasting on a grain spill next to a farmer's field, but thankfully they were off the road for the most part. Then a barn cat who was trying to play Evil Kenevil as he ran out in front of me, stopped, went 6 inches one way then back 8 inches several times before he decided which way to go.

When I finally saw the outdoor light at my friend's house, I let out an audible sigh. I couldn't wait to get out of the damn car. As I turned in her long driveway, there was 2 more stinking racoons - I kid you not. They ran into the corn field pretty fast, but at this point I actually hit my steering wheel and said out loud, "Oh come on!". As soon as my friend opened the door, she stopped mid-greeting and asked if I was ok. I proceeded to inform her about my crazy Twilight Zone drive over.

I still have no idea what natural phenomenon was taking place that night, but whatever it was, was something big. Funny thing was though that when I headed home a few hours later, I didn't see anything, not one living creature. I guess they'd had their fun and were done messing with me for the night!

Drunken Canoeing

One of the annual events back in the party days was Drunken Canoeing. Sounds like a bad idea (and it was definitely not high on the safety standards), but it was such a blast! A huge group of us would load up and drive about 4 hours into northern Michigan, USA to a campsite. The camp owners would shudder when they saw our convoy and send us up to the "Rugged Area" with no electricity or water and lots of flying, biting things. They made sure we were far, far away from the more civilized family camping. Every morning, my boyfriend at the time would start a car, stick his head out the window and yell, "All aboard the shit-house trolley!". We would stumble out of our tents in shifts and he would drive us down to the public bathrooms. After this morning routine, we would start getting packed up to head out on our favorite part of the trip. By pack up I mean your booze, your cooler floaty and a Ziploc bag of sunscreen, a bit of money and smokes. I mentioned that we were high class, right??? Then we loaded up on a rickety old school bus that was definitely NOT road worthy and were taken about 1/2 hour away to the mouth of a river.

We would go in and rent our canoes for about 10 bucks and then go back outside and wait with all the other hungover patrons. This river was perfect. It was a long, winding river with a steady but not dangerous current and was only about 5 ft deep. So, the benefit was of course there was only steering to be done, NO PADDLING. Unless you had one of those beer hats with the straw, it would have been far too hard to hold your drink AND paddle!

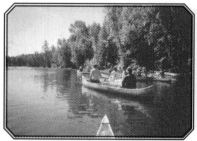

Some of the crew.

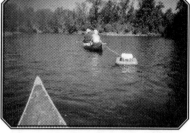

Only bring the necessities.

So, we would pair up, ungracefully board our canoe and unsuccessfully try to remain with our group. After about half an hour, everyone usually got the hang of it and had broken off into smaller, easier to maintain splinter groups. We had no life jackets but the disgusting, beat up, moldy seat pads sometimes floated, so yee-haw let's go! We would even bring bungee cords to tie the canoes together, so we could float downstream en masse or take turns jumping out to do some drunken floating (my personal favorite). An interesting point was brought to my attention by the hilarious comedian Ron White when he was recounting a similar adventure with his friends. You are out on the water for hours, drinking enough to kill a moose, but nobody ever had to pee......funny, same with our crew!

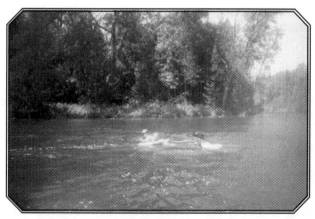

Some friends and I enjoying the lost art of drunken floating.

It would take all day to get to the pickup point on the river and the poor workers would be wading out into the water to catch the canoes that were either unmanned, had a passed-out occupant, or had someone simply too wasted to steer into shore. It was very important that we get out at the pickup point because the water got much rougher past there. The very bumpy ride back to our cars through the woods was never enjoyable and usually involved some over exuberant campers to lose their liquid lunch. The trip back to the campsite, however, on paved roads was much better and was filled with tales of the adventures of the day. We would make a big supper when we got back and then everyone would be passed out before dark (I'm sure all the other campers in the park appreciated that).

Sometimes we would pack up the next day and sometimes stay just to camp. Needless to say, by the end of the trip we were tired, hung-over, sunburnt and smelled like hot dog cooler water (only water available to wash up with). But man, were we happy and already planning the next year's visit!

Public Service Announcement

I decided to include this short story not because it's a great story but because it is one of those things that needs to be shared in the interest of public safety. I was stunned when I heard what happened, because it's something we've ALL done and never given a second thought to.

While working at the dairy practice, we received a frantic phone call about our hospital manager's husband being in an accident. The manager took the day off and when she came back the following day, she told us the story. Her husband had been volunteering at a charity BBQ and once everything was set up and ready, he was asked to loosen all the ketchup lids (it was a senior's luncheon). He happily started going through the case of ketchup and one by one picking each one up and smacking it on the bottom of the glass jar to loosen the seal, then twisting off the lid. He continued doing this robotically while chatting with the other volunteers. Then all hell broke loose. He smacked one bottle, it shattered, and he drove several pieces of glass directly through his hand! Holy shit. He ended up doing massive damage to his hand (severed tendons, etc). The worst part for him was that he was a transport truck driver and was unable to work because that was his shifting hand.

Like I said, not a great or entertaining story, but considering how many times I've smacked the bottom of a glass bottle (and been lucky) I wanted to let everyone know the dark side of bottle spanking!

Boz

I have always been obsessed with Irish Wolfhounds since I was 6 years old and saw my first one. I was adamant that one day I would have one, but just as adamant that I would never buy any dog as long as there are millions of unwanted dogs dying in shelters every year. Every one of my eight dogs and three cats have been rescues. I was very surprised to find a crossbreed because most breeders have people sign a no-breeding contract. Well Boz's story was that Mom (Irish Wolfhound) was contained by a 6ft chain link fence so Dad must have been an incredibly athletic Romeo, who climbed that fence, romanced mom and climbed back out.

I received a frantic call from Annabel one day that I couldn't understand because she was talking so fast and had almost reached a level that only dogs and bats could hear (fairly normal occurrence for her). When she finally calmed down, she told me (again) that she had found the perfect dog for me. You see, I had been without a dog for several months since my last one had passed away. I tried to explain that I didn't think I was ready yet, and she cut me off stating emphatically that this was MY dog. She told me that he was a huge Irish Wolfhound cross, very sweet but needed a lot of work and had me written all over him. The previous owners were giving him away because, get this, he got too big. I have heard a lot of stupid excuses for abandoning your dog through all my years in clinics and shelters, but this is one of my most hated ones. You went and saw the puppies. You went and saw the mother who was an Irish Wolfhound (one of the largest dogs in the world). You picked the biggest puppy. What the hell did you think he was going to grow into, a fucking Chihuahua????!!!!

Anyways, it got worse. He wasn't trained. He wasn't neutered. He lived in a townhouse with a miniscule backyard. He didn't go on walks because he was "too strong". He didn't travel well in a car. He was very mouthy (not biting but using his mouth inappropriately on people's hands/arms). But the best was yet to come. So, against my better judgement, I agreed to go meet him. All the way there I kept repeating, "I will NOT take him home. I will NOT take him home." You already know how that turned out.

I came in the front door and he came barreling in the back door right up to me, tongue hanging out, tail wagging and gave me his paw - I was screwed. Knowing full well that he was mine, I talked to the dingdongs for a little bit and told them I had to think about it overnight (ya right). As I was leaving she says, "Sorry he was so wound up, but my husband was just out playing police dog with him". Dramatic pause. "Excuse me?" "Oh, don't worry, he loves it! My husband puts on 2 winter coats and the dog chases him and grabs him by the arm, just like a police dog!" "So, you have actually trained a 120lb (was very underweight at the time), unneutered male dog with zero manners how to bite people and tackle them to the ground??" "Yes! Isn't it cool?"

Sweet lord in heaven, now I had heard everything. I left there with my head spinning. So, the next day I called her and said I would take him, because he needed to get the hell out of there and apparently, I felt I needed a HUGE problem dog challenge in my already busy life. I told her they could drop him off in a week because I had a lot going on that week and wanted to give him my undivided attention. She agreed.

Five days later I got a call from her asking if I could get him early. "Not really, why?" "Oh, because we moved the day after you were here, and he's been living in the empty townhouse all alone!!" WTF? WTF? WTF? You have got to be kidding me! Am I on Punked? Needless to say, he did not live there any longer. Here's some stories about my favorite dog.

*   *   *   *   *

One of our favorite places to go for a walk was on a path through a wooded area that used to be train tracks. I would use a 20ft horse lunge line, so he could have freedom to snoop around and be a dog. One fateful day, that generosity bit me in the ass.

I was talking on my cell phone (mistake #1) to my ex-boyfriend (mistake #2). Boz had lagged behind me to sniff something disgusting and I kept going (mistake #3). Suddenly, a blur of fur raced by me at lightning speed. Too late, I realized what was about to happen, once I too, saw the damn rabbit. Frantically, I attempted to remove my wrist from the lead....even while I was launched into the air. My cell phone went flying almost as far as I did.......and landed much more gracefully. With my right arm at full extension, I came down HARD on the GRAVEL trail and then was dragged until he realized there was a problem. Then he cheerfully ran back to me and gave me dozens of kisses. (Did you see it mom?? Did you? Did you? Did you see the bunny??") I got up very slowly, sure that something was broken and was relieved to be all in one piece. I found my broken cell phone. I wound up the long line. The adrenaline started to wear off and the pain started to register....and the blood started flowing freely.

Knowing that my analytical self would want to know later, I quickly and roughly measured the distance of my flight and crash landing by pacing them out from the clearly defined departure point, landing, skid and blessed end. I was completely airborne for about 9 feet and was dragged in the gravel for about 10 feet.

After noting the distances and suppressing the urge to send the big galoot to Alcatraz, I started assessing our injuries.

Boz - 100% totally fine. I honestly don't even think he realized what had happened until the gravel pile that my limp body was pushing got too heavy to pull.

Me
- road rash/cheese grater type injuries to my head, neck, entire right arm, armpit, right boob, ribcage, hip, knee and ankle
- goose egg forming on side of my head
- large chunks of gravel stuck in arm and armpit and boob
- right palm of hand resembling raw hamburger.
- broken sunglasses, broken phone
- blood everywhere
- ripped shirt

Now for the good news, we still had a 4 1/2 km walk back home!! I must have been emitting some pretty serious, "don't mess with me" vibes, because that big mutt was as obedient as a guide dog and the half dozen people we passed gave me a wide berth and strange looks. (thinking about it now though, why the hell didn't anyone ask if I was OK??)

Anyways, we made it home, I got cleaned up, used a whole box of Band-Aids and a whole tube of Polysporin after using my tweezers to remove copious gravel fragments from my arm, armpit and boob. I wrapped my hand (which was actually the worst part) and did my best to clean up my head. I called the ex back to let him know I was alive (in hindsight, I should have just faked my own death and been done with that mess!) Then I sat down and had a beer.

Lesson for today?? Don't let a 140lb (he was now at a proper weight) dog with longer legs than yours get a 40 foot running head start while you are attached. Funny thing is that being a horse lover, I know you never wrap a horse line for exactly that reason but clearly, I didn't use that same logic with my big boy. My fault, not his. But the worst part is that he never even caught the damn rabbit after all that!

Oh well, he more than made up for this day in the years to come.

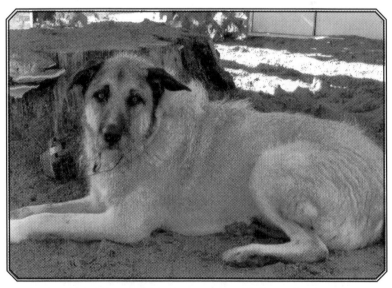

Best pic I have of his famous 6-inch-long foo-man-choo beard because it was usually cut off due to his incredible talent of finding burrs with it.

Boz and The Boz

As I said, my infatuation with Irish Wolfhounds began early at the age of 6 when I saw my first one. I was awestruck by their size, beauty, gracefulness and regal presence.

My infatuation with Brian Bosworth began at the age of 13 when I first saw him. I was awestruck by the size of his muscles, his handsomeness and his hubba hubba factor. I devoured anything I could to learn about him and his football career (I didn't follow football at the time). I bought all his movies (on VHS). I got an autographed jersey of my beloved #44. I read his autobiography, bought pictures, magazines, trading cards, you name it. I can still recite all the lines of Stone Cold (his best movie) with over a 90% success rate........OK, maybe that was TMI...I'm starting to sound like a stalker! I remember a few stories where my appreciation of this fine individual caused me to make a bit of a scene...or 2.

*   *   *   *   *

I was at a bar with a bunch of college buddies enjoying some pizza and some pitchers one night when suddenly the TV caught my eye. I froze with my beer 1/2way to my mouth. After a few seconds my friends noticed my weird behaviour and they were concerned that I was choking on something. Then my boyfriend followed my gaze and started laughing, saying,

"She's ok! Don't worry, she's just gone into a Brian Bosworth coma! Get me the remote control stat!"

Everyone roared, except a couple people who inevitably asked the question, "Who is he?".

"Oh hell, don't ask her THAT!" he complained.

I snapped out of it and proceeded to regale them with stories and information until several hands were placed over my mouth! I sat staring at the TV for the next few hours by myself watching the launch of the XFL, which Mr. Bosworth happened to be one of the commentators for. I had a renewed interest in football suddenly.

*   *   *   *   *

Many years later, my friends and I were going to see the remake of the Longest Yard in the theatre. We were looking forward to it even though we hadn't heard too much about it other than it had Adam Sandler and a bunch of wrestlers in it. (and yes, in case you're wondering, I followed WWE for many years and No, I'm not embarrassed about it! Where else do you get to see so many handsome, buff men?)

So as the movie starts the patrons quiet down and we watched about 10 minutes happily munching on our chemically altered popcorn with "butter-like topping" - I mean really, how expensive is butter for heaven's sake?? Then the prison bus scene begins and where my sanity ended.

"Holy shit! That's Brian Bosworth! Did you see? That's him! Did you know he was in this? Why didn't you tell me? It's Brian Bosworth!" Only at the end of my outburst did I realize that I was standing. And that several people were staring at me and several more were "shushing me". I sat down unfazed (I can't say the same for my friends!) and watched the rest of the movie with the rabid attention of a bomb squad diffusing napalm.

The point of embarrassing myself by telling you these stories is so you understand the significance and importance of the name. Brian Bosworth used to go by the name "The Boz" back in the day (in case any of you have the audacity not to know that already...shame on you!). He was also a linebacker. I always said that when I finally got a dog the size of a linebacker, I would bestow upon him the highest honor and let him be known as Bosworth....and so it was.

*   *   *   *   *

During our first week together, I learned a lot about him. I discovered that he had no idea how big he was, he thought he was a lap dog (as most XL dogs do) and his favorite place to sit was backing up on my lap while his front feet stayed on the floor. This made any movement on my part very difficult and if I dared struggle or shift, he would look back at me, sigh and push his big butt down harder!

I also learned that he was unable/unwilling to make quick decisions. For example, we were playing fetch in my big backyard which he loved because it finally gave him a chance to stretch those ridiculously long legs. I was caught up in the moment, beautiful day, new best friend, dog of my dreams, watching him gracefully gallop in great strides....right at me....he'll stop....he'll swerve....he'll ......BANG! His decision was to run directly into my thighs/hips at full speed with his head. After impact I flew up and did a very sloppy front somersault IN THE AIR and landed flat on my back, knocking the wind out of me. I felt like I'd been hit by a dump truck. He came right over, stood over me looking down, very confused, as if to say, "What 'cha doing down there??" As I looked up at him, catching my breath, I couldn't help but laugh. I couldn't have picked a better name for my linebacker!

*   *   *   *   *

When I brought my son home from the hospital, poor ol' Boz didn't know what to make of him. He was beyond thrilled to have me home, but unsure of this little screaming thing attached to me. He was very curious but had a very low tolerance for the crying and would ask to be let outside soon after any fussing began.

I was very "on the ball" about my son's safety and my dog's well being (even in my new-mom-sleep-deprived state) and it was always in my mind about how they would interact as they got older. Boz never exhibited any worrisome behaviour but didn't show a whole lot of interest either. New mom brain had me overanalyzing and worrying since my bond with Boz was like nothing I had ever experienced before, and I wanted my son to experience the same amazing feeling.

One day when my son was about 8 months old, I had him outside on a blanket with me in the shade of a huge tree. Boz was about 20ft away laying in the sun. After awhile he got up and walked slowly over, sniffed my son and laid down near him, propped up on his elbows and on alert. I cried. Quietly. I didn't want to ruin this beautiful moment that I had waited so long for. I was so incredibly thankful. Boz made such a powerful statement with such a simple gesture. He had finally welcomed Jake into our family and officially appointed himself as Jake's protector. He carried out his promise until the day he died.

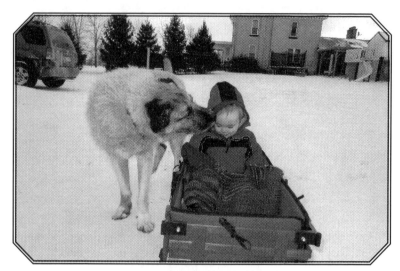

The loves of my life.

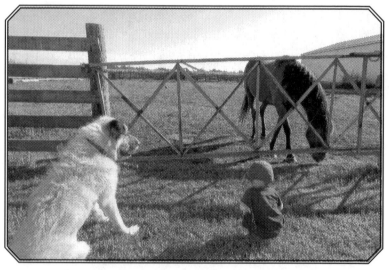

Boz NEVER let my son get close to my horse.
He would stand guard like this and then put his
body in between them if my son moved.

Therefore, it was no surprise and a fitting tribute when Jake's first words at 11 months were Boz's name. Not Boz exactly but "Gig Bob". At the time, my ex's dog was living there too, and she was a sweet little 40lb girl, Boz was a 140lb boy, so for simplicity we referred to them as "Little Dog" and "Big Dog" for Jake. Boz came into the living room one day and Jake excitedly pointed at him and said, "Gig Bob! Gig Bob!" I was thrilled!

Gig Bob, Big Dog, Boz, my love, our protector, my heartfelt thanks.

*   *   *   *   *

When people would be nervous or scared of Boz because of his size, I would always tell them what a sweet, friendly boy he was. I would also tell them that as long as I was happy, Boz was happy. Most dogs pick up on their owners' moods, but he was exceptionally good at it. We had gotten in a few situations where I was a little uncomfortable (going for walks at night, running into shady characters) and without any big production Boz would stand taller, widen his shoulders and put himself between me and the "bad guy". He never once growled or bared his teeth - he didn't need to. His calm, uber-confident stature was more than enough to discourage any wrong doing. He would just make his presence known and carry on being my personal body guard until I was at ease, then he would return to his big goofy self instantly.

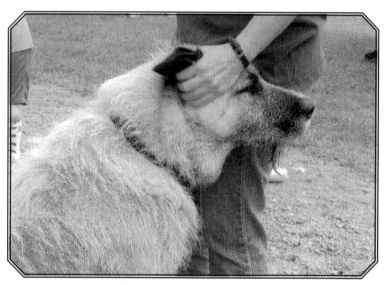

Boz and I routinely traded ear massages for being the eyes in the back of my head. I have never felt so safe and protected in all my life then when I was with Boz.

There was one time that the body guarding went a little too far. We were having a neighbourhood pot luck supper with lots of people. A boyfriend of one of the teenagers was making the rounds hugging the ladies and thanking us for the meal because they were leaving. When he got to me, he hugged me, lifted me up a bit and then froze (with me up). The room roared with laughter and I didn't know what was going on. He let go of me and Boz let go of his butt cheek! Let me be clear - this was not a bite, this was Boz making a point the only way he knew how when the "attacker" couldn't see him posturing. He didn't break the skin, didn't tear the pants, he merely held on to the poor kid's ass until he let me go! Once I was free, he non-chalantly sauntered away a few feet and plopped down to go back to sleep. Needless to say, I didn't' get any more hugs that night.

* * * * *

One night after Jake was asleep, Boz jumped up and whined at the door with urgency. He had some stomach trouble in his last year, so I just assumed it was nature calling. As I opened the door, I realized too late that it WAS nature calling - a pack of coyotes, very close. Boz took off like greased lightning (when he ran full out, he had over a 2m stride). The coyotes were about 300ft away behind the big drive shed and as Boz rounded the corner their howls and yips changed immediately to yelps and barks (imagine their surprise) I was so worried. Boz was easily big enough and tough enough to take on probably 3-4 coyotes, but not a whole pack. Thankfully my landlord was right next door having a boys night in his shop, so I burst in, in my pajamas screaming, "Get your gun!". All the local fellas looked up, eyes wide, beers 1/2 tipped to open mouths (imagine THEIR surprise!). I didn't' care, I ran out into the night as far as my baby monitor's reception would go. The coyotes were way back in the bush now, very riled up and noisy. My heart sank. Did they get him?? I headed back to the shop to get the men to watch the baby monitor, so I could go looking for my Boz.

The landlord met me outside with his gun. I told him all that had happened so far. As we were figuring out a plan what to do next, I heard something behind the corn dryers. It was Boz! My heart leapt out of my chest. As I was running to him, I had to stop and laugh. He was limping slightly but had a hugely satisfied look on his face and a cocky swagger to his step. He looked like a drunk guy who just won a bar fight!

I dropped to my knees, gave him a huge hug and kisses and then proceeded to give him shit, "Don't you EVER do that again! I was worried sick!" (well, I am a mom now). Doug went back to his boys night, even though he'd sobered up from all the excitement, and Boz and I went back in the house. He got many treats and thank yous and love and one more half-hearted scolding :)

There's not too many dogs that can single handedly run off a large pack of coyotes and live to tell about it, but I'm sure glad he was able to have bragging rights.

*　　*　　*　　*　　*

Boz was also very effective pest control on the farm. No squirrel, rabbit, muskrat, rat, raccoon or SKUNK was safe. I have spent many pages telling you how amazing and smart and wonderful Boz was. Now for his downfall. SIX, I repeat, SIX skunks were killed, ripped apart and rolled in, in less than 2 years. For an animal that has a nose 50 000 times better than ours you'd think they would learn after the first spray, but alas, these stinky critters were Boz's Achilles heel. He even got 2 of them in the dead of winter when they should be hibernating. He became the neighbourhood joke whenever that distinct odor would waft around the area, "Boz got another one!"

I went through litres of skunk shampoo in that time period and he had to sleep in the barn a few times (much to my grumpy horse's dismay) but even his weakness for skunks couldn't tarnish his gold medal standing in my heart.

*　　*　　*　　*　　*

Less stinky, but more surprising for me was when I lived on a 50-acre farm with him. Most of the acreage was bush and I walked him through it regularly. One day he was acting really wired/on the hunt and as I worried he was after a skunk, he flushed out a baby deer!! Tiny little thing but man could it move! It definitely "one-upped" the big guy for manoeuvrability through the dense brush. I started running after them, yelling for Boz to stop, leave it and come back. I mean, who could live with themselves if they had anything to do with killing Bambi? As I ran, I heard/

saw some activity in the bushes in front of me, so I stopped and started praising him for coming back. That's when Mama leapt out of the bush and landed within 2 ft of me! We both froze, pupils dilated for 3-4 seconds. I literally could have reached out and touched her. Just as suddenly as she appeared, she vanished into the woods and very soon after Boz came running back, limping and exhausted, but happy. I'll never know what happened, but my guess is that Mama tuned him in for chasing her baby (and rightly so).

Not to worry, I saw Mama and baby a few days later drinking out of our pond behind the house and both appeared fine. I knew it was her because she was the most beautiful colour I'd ever seen, not a normal deer colour. She was a solid, dark coppery red - just stunning. I was blown away at how beautiful and big she was up close and I'm very grateful that she didn't kick the crap out of me. As thanks to her, I made it a habit to be excessively noisy as we entered the bush from then on. Boz didn't appreciate it and would actually stop and look back at me like, "Hellooooo? I'm trying to hunt here do you mind??"

*   *   *   *   *

I could go on and on about Boz because my heart just bursts with love, fond memories and laughter when I think about him. My eyes also stream with tears and I still get so sad and angry that he's gone. I rescued him when he was 3 years old and he rescued me for the next 7 years.

Forever in my heart and my memories. You were one of a kind and will be remembered by all that had the privilege of meeting you. May you always live on in my words. RIP big fella.

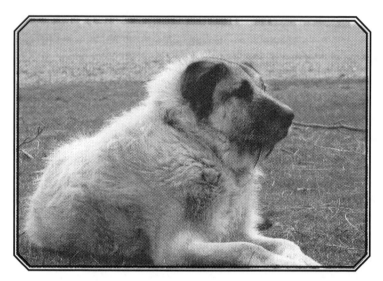

Forever in my heart.

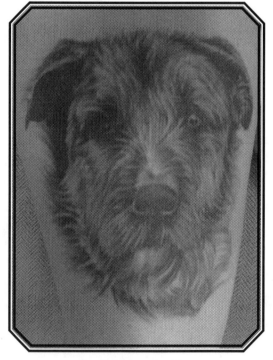

Forever in my skin.

CRUE

Being a hardcore headbanger since the age of 12, I have many stories dealing with concerts, but the best ones deal with Motley Crue.

Around the age of 25, a van-full of us drove to Toronto to see their show. I had walking pneumonia. I shouldn't have been anywhere except a hospital bed, but youth and stupidity are powerful forces that can slay common sense in the blink of an eye. I don't remember ever being so sick, but apparently being crushed by 10,000 other people surrounded by cigarette and pot smoke, blaring music and pyrotechnics was too hard to pass up.

When we first got there, we were trying to make our way to our seats and as I was pushing my way through the crowd, I launched into a massive coughing spell which dislodged about 6 pounds of gunk from my lungs. That would have been bad enough on its own, but the last cough completely emptied my lungs of air and the sticky gunk then formed an impenetrable seal over my windpipe. I couldn't breathe in and I had no air left to cough out. I frantically shoved my way through the crowd like a linebacker. I started seeing stars and getting ready to collapse. Thankfully my friend followed me (thinking I was heading somewhere good) and when I doubled over clutching a railing for support, she took one look at my purple face started beating the hell out of my back. Luckily her pummeling was able to loosen a tiny bit of the gunk and I was able to suck in some air. It felt like I was breathing through a juice box straw but at least I was breathing! After several looooooong minutes, I was able to get enough air to cough hard enough to dislodge the crud, stop the room from spinning and stand up. So, at this point a logical person would call it a night and go home right?? Haha! Not a chance! We stayed for the whole thing, drove 3 hours back home (where I promptly fell into bed and didn't move for 3 days)

A couple years later the same friend and I went to an outdoor Crue show and I was in perfect health! She on the other hand, was dealing with some pretty big anxiety issues concerning the large crowd and lack of structure (no seating, open field). We found an area that wasn't too packed, well away from the pit and she was doing great until a huge thunderstorm hit, complete with massive bolts of lightning. This is perhaps a good time to inform you that her absolute biggest fears are severe weather, large crowds and jellyfish. I was pretty sure we were safe on the last fear but the other two were definitely front and center! The poor girl turned bone white, started shaking and was on the verge of tears. She tried to stick it out, but after a couple minutes it was way too much for her and we started to head out. Keep in mind though that this was no easy task pushing through tons of people slipping in mud and avoiding lightning and mosh pits!

Once we finally made it back to the car, she felt much better, but then started to feel guilty about me not seeing the whole show. I just laughed and said, "If it hadn't been for you at the last Crue show I would have died! The least I can do for you is leave a bit early for you!"

In 2014 Crue had their farewell tour and of course Lungbutter and Lightning just had to go. It was a great time and NOTHING bad happened – we were shocked!

Pulled Over

Luckily, I have not had a lot of experience being pulled over. Besides routine RIDE programs, it's only happened once, when I lived in a teeny little, rural town.

I was leaving a house call where I was checking up on a German Shepherd who had recently whelped a very large litter. She was on IV fluids at home and several medications due to birthing complications. Normally, she would have been kept at the animal hospital but due to the pups and her stress we decided to leave her at home with regular daily checkups. As I was driving back to the clinic, I went through a strange little 1km area where it's 90km/hr at the top of the hill, 50km/hr at the bottom and then 90 again heading back up the other side. You see where this is heading. The cherries flipped on (simultaneously with my potty mouth) and I pulled over.

This very young cop (keep in mind, I was only in my early 20's at the time and he still looked young!) who was obviously nervous and unsure did his very best attempt at being confident and authoritative. I got my license and insurance out and tried to hand them over - but he wasn't looking at me. His gaze was steadily fixed to the very large box of syringes, needles, drugs and bloody gloves in the passenger seat beside me. I'd forgotten all about it!

Looking like he was going to implode at any moment I smiled and spoke very calmly and softly. I explained who I was, what my job was, where I was coming from and where I was going. He finally looked at me slightly stunned. I opened my winter coat, so he could see my scrubs and the RVT embroidered on my shirt. I offered the clinic's phone number and said he could follow me to work and speak to my boss. He stumbled and stuttered over his words but said he would follow me back. He turned to go back to his car, then stopped, came back and gave me a ticket for speeding! Are you serious? I just gave you some on the job training! I handled you with kid gloves! I...oh screw it, I was doing 95 in a 50 (however stupid the teeny-weeny bottom of the hill 50km/hr was). He did follow me back but never came in the clinic. Oh well, at least I gave that rookie a good story to share when he got back to the station!

Wanita, Jeff and Brenda

So, this crazy lady came into my life through my ex that defies explanation. She's amazing, eccentric, hilarious and intelligent. Since meeting her several years ago, we have developed a unique and wicked friendship that is a strict no B.S. zone. We share the same twisted sense of humor, the same ways of dealing with people and situations and the same attitude all while being different enough to complement each other beautifully and provide intelligent, enjoyable, entertaining conversation that has yet to last less than 2 hours/phone call.

Needless to say, I was thrilled when she said she was coming to visit me in the hospital. Upon her arrival, she presented me with a cute little purple box and said she knew how much I missed the outdoors, so she brought it inside to me. Super sweet, super thoughtful thing to do! As I started going through the box, she excused herself to go to the washroom. There were pine needles, leaves, pretty tiny flowers, small stones, a pine cone....what the hell???? WANITA!!!!

She came flying out of the bathroom just in time to catch the box that I was about to hurl across the room. She looked genuinely shocked. All I could say was, "Spiders!". She looked in, started laughing and kept repeating "Sorry!" through her laughter. Apparently attached to one of her gifts must have been a nest of spiders that conveniently hatched on her drive to the hospital and were taking over the box!

Once I frantically checked my bedding and body for the 11th time, I relaxed and saw the humor in the situation and we both laughed till exhaustion. Only Wanita would have brought a box full of friggin' spiders to an arachnophobe on bed rest!

*   *   *   *   *

Another close friend of mine, Jeffery, also made a memorable impact on my time in the hospital (minus the spiders). He had battled OCD and pretty severe anxiety his whole life and it really impacted him. I knew he wanted to support me and help however he could, but I also knew that driving on the highway and in big cities were 2 of his worst triggers. He didn't like new places or large crowds either. The hospital I was in was huge, it was on the biggest intersection of the city which had a population of 350 000. We talked on the phone and he had promised to try and come visit. I appreciated his offer, but I just knew he wouldn't be able to come. But I came back from one of my multitudes of tests/procedures one day and lo and behold - there he was! I was stunned. We had a great visit and I was so appreciative that he would go to such lengths for me! His strength was inspiring.

*   *   *   *   *

Yet another wonderful person who gave me some smiles was Beth, a friend of Diane's who just happened to be an ICU nurse in that same hospital. She wasn't on my floor, but she made several late-night junk food drop offs for me on her way to work and would stay and chat with me for a bit each time. We only knew each other through Diane but she still took the time and made the effort to help me out. Her thoughtfulness and concern for someone she didn't even know that well spoke volumes of her character and the size of her heart.

Evil

I adopted a small tortoiseshell kitten from one of the clinics I worked at. She was hell on wheels, as most torti's are. I named her Mayhem, but my ex nicknamed her "The Runt" because she was so tiny, and it stuck until a few years later when "Evil" became her moniker (for good reason).

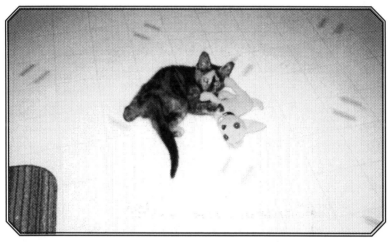

Taco dog getting his butt kicked.

When she was about 3 months old, she displayed her true colours in an amazing show of attitude and arrogance (while weighing in at a whopping 2.5lbs). I was laying on the couch watching TV and she was across the room sitting on an end table. She swatted over a framed picture, so I said firmly, "Hey! Quit it!". She stopped, stared at me, casually jumped down, walked across the room, jumped up on me, stared at me again and swatted me in the face! I was in shock. She then proceeded to walk back across the room, jump on the table and knock over another picture!

I laughed for 15 minutes straight. I've never been much of a cat person, which is why it surprised me that I even adopted her, but I loved her "spark" and this little turd was proving to be my kind of girl.

She also used to puff up and walk very slowly and directly to the door when someone knocked, while making short, punctuated growl/bark noises. She would have gone viral for sure nowadays!

*   *   *   *   *

One of my favorite Evil stories took place at a house I was living at with her, another special cat and 2 large dogs. It was a well-established rule that there was no running/rough housing in the house so when my big shepherd X came tearing through the living room at Mach 9 one day, I was quite surprised. Even more surprised when he continued doing donuts through the main floor while completely ignoring me (he was incredibly obedient). I let out a guttural yell that cut through his apparent brain fog and let him know I meant business (I had never raised my voice like that with him before, but this situation was nuts). He literally skidded to a stop like a reining horse and sat there shaking and panting and drooling a few feet away.   As I headed over to see what the hell just happened, I immediately found the problem.......attached to his neck!

Apparently my 90lb dog had crossed some sort of line with my 7lb cat. In order to resolve the situation Evil had decided to embed her teeth and all 4 paws full of nails into and around the dog's throat and neck. She continued her assault all the way down the stairs and for at least 4-5 laps around the main floor and had still not let go!

I rushed over and removed the demonic troll from my poor dogs' neck. He quickly ran to the back door, begging to be let outside to get away from his assailant. My other dog was already at the door with a panicked look in his eyes. I let the dogs out and looked down at Evil, who was still in my arms and casually grooming herself and purring. I just laughed, set her down and went out to check for damage on my big tough dog. After calming him down and examining his physical wounds I tried to bring him back in the house, only to realize his emotional wounds were far more severe! He took one look at that tiny terror sitting on the counter and put the brakes on. He did come in later that day but both dogs remained on high alert whenever she entered the room for the rest of their lives. Thankfully, there was never another altercation with those boys.

I still wonder what the hell happened that day. Just goes to show the old saying is true "It's not the size of the dog (or cat) in the fight, it's the size of the fight in the dog (or cat)".

PS. If anyone is wondering why I couldn't see her on him initially, it's because he was mostly black with brindle and a shaggy mane and she was a tiny cat with torti markings. Their colours blended beautifully, even if their personalities didn't!

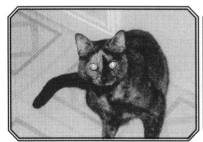

The assailant.

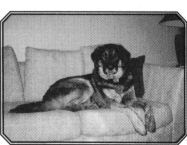

The victim.

Earring

While working in a very small rural dairy veterinary clinic I had an interesting experience. For those unfamiliar with bovine surgery, I will briefly explain. Most surgery on cattle is done while they are standing. They are sedated and have local anesthetic, so they are as comfy as possible but standing. My job as the tech was to prepare for surgery (instruments, drapes, medications) prepare the animal (sedate, clip the area, prep area and inject local freezing) then to assist the DVM and recover the animal afterwards.

We were getting ready to do a C-section on a very large Hereford cow and everything was going along tickety-boo. The doctor made his incision, which is necessarily large for the big baby about to come out. Once he incised the uterus, my job was to go into her abdomen with both hands/arms (which had been sterily scrubbed) and hold onto it with everything I had. It is a HUGE muscle that is actively contracting and trying to disappear back into her equally huge body as soon as the baby is removed safely. In this particular cow, the uterus was ridiculous. I felt like I was being pulled right in! The bull calf was enormous and being attended to by the other staff (and doing well).

My hands and arm muscles were screaming for a break, but you just CAN'T let go or the Dr is left searching through an abdomen the size of a small car for a bleeding organ and the poor cow would be up the proverbial creek without a paddle. As always, when your hands are occupied, I got a terrible itch on my face. I fought to ignore it for a while but then caved and put one knee up against the cow for balance and used my left shoulder for rub my face. Relief! Until....2 seconds after solving the itch, I watched in horror as one of my small silver earrings rolled down my arm into the open incision and disappeared INTO the cow! As my jaw hit my chest, I looked up at the DVM and his eyes were the size of dinner plates! I suddenly forgot about my aching arms as he called for more light and proceeded to do as in depth a search as humanly possible. After a few minutes he gave up and continued to stitch up her uterus, muscle wall and skin. Stopping all the bleeding and finishing surgery before freezing wore off and reuniting her with her calf were far more important.

Thankfully the cow did amazingly well and went on to have several more babies with no side effects from her very strange, very small foreign body. Of course, we were honest with the farmer and he just laughed, brushed it off and said something to the effect of "Next time I eat at McDonald's I'll just chew slowly so I don't chip a tooth!"

Best Day Ever

In 2005 I had the best day ever. My dad and I went on a trip to Daytona, Florida for Bike Week. We spent days touring the thousands upon thousands of bikes. Some of them were mind-bogglingly cool. We had a great time, but the best was yet to come.

I was lucky enough to spend a whole day at Discovery Cove, taking part in their "Trainer for a Day" program. The day started early, and we had to be at the park before 7am. I got fitted in a wetsuit and broke off into small groups of 6 with one staff member. From there we spent the whole day experiencing the park. That day, the temperature was only about 50 degrees and in true Canadian style, I wore a flannel jacket over my wetsuit (sexy beast)! We started by seeing and feeding a plethora of tropical, free flying birds. Nice. Then moved on to feeding a bunch of sharks with a long pole. Scary but cool. I don't know what kind they were but do know that there was no rail around the pool and there was some in the tank that were bigger than me. Eeeek.

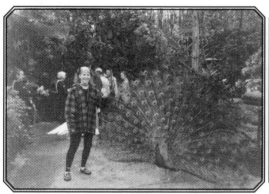
Sexy beast.

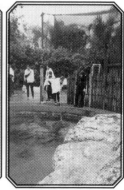
I think we need a bigger pole.

Then we got a pouch of slimy, gross little fish and were told how to hold them to feed a huge pool of stingrays without getting our fingers crushed off. My excitement got me in the waist-deep water first and for a fraction of a second, I regretted it. I was literally swarmed by dozens of rays all jostling for position and I literally had to fight for balance! They would flip up sideways against my body, trying to get their mouths (on their underside) close to the food. Then they got pissy because apparently, I was too slow and they'd start slapping me with their fin that was out of the water. I've been in my share of tussles, but I've never been "bitch slapped" by a sea creature before! I was laughing my ass off, but the dry participants were not sharing my excitement - only 2 others eventually came in to join me while the other 3 stayed on dry land with wide eyes. I had to keep reminding myself to keep all my digits tucked into a fist, so the rays didn't mistake my fingers for fish and suck them in and crush them with their powerful back teeth. This was harder than it seems though because they were very strong, large, slippery and determined to get pole position and I almost lost my balance several times. It was definitely a unique and crazy experience and I was able to do it for a long time because the other people let me have their pouches of gooey fish since they weren't coming in - awesome!

Next, we sat through a few videos and an info session for the big event. I was vibrating with excitement and it seemed to take forever. To add insult to injury, we were then told to go have lunch. Lunch?? Who could eat at a time like this?? I went and found my dad who only had a general admission (poor guy) and had a few bites to eat while I prattled on about my morning. He didn't get 2 words in then I bolted back to rejoin the group. I'm pretty sure at this point, he found a bench and had a nap.

We entered the huge pool. Out of the depths, she emerged like magic and time stood still. I was chest deep in water, 2 feet away from a dolphin. Her name was Latoya and she was unequivocally the most amazing, beautiful creature I'd ever seen. The trainer was saying lots of things that I'm sure were very interesting and important, but nothing short of my hair catching fire could have shifted my focus. I had the most surreal feeling of exhilaration and peace all at the same time. Then it was my turn to meet her (does it get any better than this?? Oh wait, it does!!)

She was floating effortlessly with her perpetual dolphin grin as I approached. With robot precision I placed my hands delicately on her where I was instructed, almost afraid that the physical contact would make this otherworldly experience disappear into thin air like a dream. I touched her, she looked directly into my eyes. There are no words. I have NEVER felt anything remotely close to that in my whole life. I was able to spend several more minutes with her and I will be eternally grateful for my experience with her. I don't know much about metaphysical stuff or energy stuff or even voodoo for that matter, but SOMETHING happened that day! After Latoya swam back to her buddies, we went on a tour of the dolphin kitchen and met some more trainers.

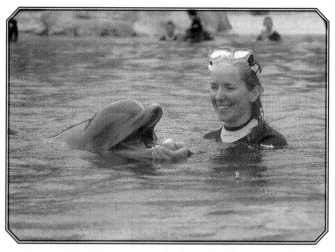

Blissed out me and Latoya.

We each got a bucket of fish and went to a big communal pool and the dolphins came over voluntarily and started showing off for us. We were able to learn a few hand signals for specific behaviours and the dolphins were more than happy to oblige. They reminded me of a bunch of kindergarten kids - watch me! watch me! Look what I can do! Wasn't that great? I can jump higher than that guy! It was hilarious, and I was surprised to see that when our buckets were empty, most of the dolphins stuck around and continued their antics for the sheer pleasure of it with only our reactions and petting as rewards. It was out of this world!

The leader then said that the day was coming to an end - what?? How did that happen? She said she had one more surprise for us. We headed back over to the huge pool where I had met Latoya and at this point 2 of the people in our group tapped out saying they were too cold. WTF? Are you shitting me?? I would have gladly chipped icicles of my flippin' nose to have this experience. To be honest, I hadn't even noticed the temperature in the last 4 hours since lunch. Oh well, their loss. The leader proceeded to go through a bunch of legal mumbo jumbo and health restrictions for the next event. I didn't care, unless they were throwing me in the shark tank, I was game for anything. I volunteered to go first. She said to follow her to the middle of the pool. "Pool" is a bit of a misleader, this body of water was huge and when you got out to the middle, the water was quite dark. She instructed me to stay afloat, but with as little movement as possible and to stay calm (DID they put me in the shark tank??). All of a sudden, she blew her whistle and these 2 HUGE bodies surfaced on either side of me. They were right below me the whole time and I didn't even know it! She introduced them as Rascal and Diego and said they were young males who were kind of shit disturbers and this was their absolute favorite thing to do. I held on to each dorsal fin and felt the immense power of the incredible animals.

They were squeaking and bumping my legs in anticipation. She asked if I was ready. I nodded, and those buggers took off at approximately 200mph. They pulled me about 250 ft and I almost blacked out from exhilaration. The speed, the power, the agility, the fun! As soon as I let go, they flipped around and dove and I kid you not they were back at the starting line in 2-3 seconds, where they started squeaking and splashing eagerly awaiting the next rider. Though I was EXTREMELY sad that the day was ending, it was still a hell of a send off.

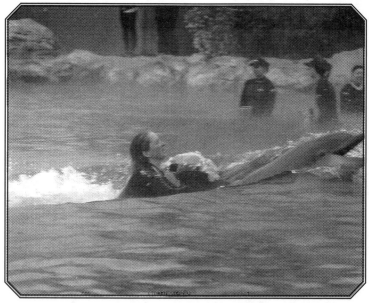

Check out the wake behind me! Yeehaw!

We were then released from our group, thank yous and good byes were said, and the trainers went off to tuck the dolphins in for the night. We were told we had about an hour left before the park closed and we could go swim in the lazy river (a 4ft deep, manmade river that wound through the park, past tropical fish, etc. Of course, I jumped in and off I swam. Not realizing how far away the change rooms were. By the time I got there, I could barely move. There was no one else in the change room. Strange. I got under the hot shower water and suddenly realized how utterly exhausted, bone crushingly sore and friggin' freezing I was. My adrenaline extravaganza was over and coming out of it was like getting hit by a semi truck. As I warmed up, I smiled and tried to get out of my wetsuit. Not going well. Tried again, fail#2. Park PA system goes off saying the park is closing in 5 minutes. Eeek! I called out for help to get the zipper unstuck but of course no one was there. I struggled, wriggled, sat on the floor and finally got out of the suit with literally my last ounces of strength and energy. "The park is now closed." echoed in my ears as I made my way to the front. I ran into my dad (the only other person there) as he looked around frantically for me, fearing I had been eaten by stingrays or something worse. I was pleasantly greeted by a "Where the hell have you been? The friggin' park is closed!" I just smiled and proceeded to regale him with all the countless stories of the day. We ate supper and I went straight to bed.

When I woke up, every muscle in my body was throbbing, my right shoulder had completely seized up and I still had a huge shit-eating grin on my face. Best day ever!

Soon after coming home I realized why they had said not to do the last ride if you had any prior back, neck or shoulder issues. My list of prior shoulder injuries included, tendonitis, bursitis, frozen shoulder twice and now (I would later find out) I had the privilege of adding 3 tears to my rotator cuff thanks to my amazing day! TOTALLY WORTH IT!

Side note: I realize that keeping wild animals in captivity is not ideal, but I also realize that having a few ambassadors in safe, stimulating environments where they are extremely well cared for, providing the general public with a chance to interact, fall in love with and become advocates for certain species also has huge benefits for the population as a whole. I have dedicated my entire life to animal welfare. I have supported the SPCA for decades. I support PBI and Sea Shepherd. I have worked in veterinary clinics, barns and shelters for 30 years. All of my pets have been rescues. I don't say any of this for any accolades, only to let the reader know that animal safety and proper treatment are paramount in my world. The animals I encountered there were happy, social, playful, well fed and the premises were clean. During our tour, we saw the entire park and there was not one shady "do not enter" area. Every dolphin had a name, they hung out in social groups and none of them were forced to work if they weren't in the mood (the trainer would just pick another one to play with for the day). Is it ideal to have captive dolphins? Of course not. But they provide a positively life altering experience for many people and appear to enjoy doing it. They give people a face to remember the next time they're asked to donate money to animal welfare or when they feel too lazy to walk their plastic waste to the recycling bin on the beach, they will think twice. To be able to connect with a magnificent creature like that changes you. One of the people in my group was an 8-year-old from "Make a Wish", her parents cried regularly that day every time they saw her laugh and smile - something she hadn't done in months. Hopefully, these dolphins sacrifice of living in captivity will benefit their species as much as they benefit ours.

Chris

I was lucky enough to have the chance to meet and become friends with the most remarkable man. Shortly after one of my many moves, I was drawn to sign up at a martial arts studio simply due to its convenient location and my desire to beat the hell out of a heavy bag (I wasn't in a yoga-zen mindset at the time) and get back in shape. The owner's name was Chris and he was a multi-discipline black belt and a hell of a guy.

We hit it off right away. The friendship felt very easy and comfortable very quickly. He adopted me as his long, lost kid sister and treated me in kind. I went to his gym 5-6 nights a week after work and my extra pounds disappeared ridiculously fast (yay!) but not easily. He was a slave driver. The thought of those workouts now makes me nauseous, especially the ones referred to as "911 workouts" where we pushed ourselves to the absolute limit and then some. But at the time, I was driven to get back in shape, the comradery in the gym was addictive and he was by far the single greatest motivator I've ever encountered. The way he could read people and what they needed was uncanny. In a class full of 16 people, he could briskly walk through the rows and change his tactics 16 times without missing a beat. He could be helping someone who'd had a bad day with positive, supportive "you can do it" stuff and then casually look over his shoulder at me, snicker and say, "my grandmother kicks harder than that!" knowing full well that my competitiveness and anger-based fire would take that snarky comment and double my efforts. Then the next day, he'd sense I was in a good/happy mood and challenge me to some sort of physical contest (handstand push ups, backwards bridge push ups, etc). He always knew how to get that extra 10% out of you that you didn't know you had but were so proud of yourself when you found it. He was also a compassionate ear many times for me and a fun, inspiring, enjoyable person to be around.

Due to no fault of his own ("It is what it is." was his favorite saying), he had to let the gym go after a couple years and he continued his teaching in his basement. A few students stayed on for awhile but eventually petered off until it was just me. He had developed a realistic, street defense system that combined many different disciplines of martial arts and was geared to women. I supported him 110% and was his guinea pig. His stuff worked. We tested and tried it repeatedly, and we were a very good representation of a worst-case scenario. He was a 6'3" 250-pound, muscular, athletic man. I was a 5'2" 120 pound, becoming athletic again woman. He had me by more than a foot and more than double my weight and the shit still worked. I couldn't wait for his big break to happen for him. While waiting for Oprah or Ellen to call him up to sit on her couch and talk about it, he busted ass trying to get it out there. We went to a large women's only gym and held classes for a group of ladies for several weeks. We were very well received, and everything went great but there was one memory from that time that will forever stay with me. There was this 50-something lady who was diminutive and terrified. I'm going to guess that she was 4'10" and 90 pounds and that someone kicked the living shit out of her, repeatedly. When she came in, she'd be shaking, pale, avoiding eye contact and hiding at the back of the room. As I said, Chris was great with people and he tried everything with her, even squatted down while talking with her but she couldn't handle it and one day even started crying. He leapt back like he'd been burned and looked at me. From then on, I worked with her, but it was like working with dynamite and having a lit smoke in your mouth. I would give her lots of warning and move very slowly (I'm going to touch your shoulder now, ok?) and she would still tremble and quiver. I have never met a braver person in my life. The balls that it took for that lady to sign up for the class and to show up every night was inconceivable. I don't know how much skill she took out of the class but just signing up for it was a huge step for her. Both Chris and I spoke repeatedly about how we would love to meet the S.O.B. who had tortured that poor thing in a dark alley with no witnesses.

Anyways, after the class Chris found a filming company that said they would make a video of his stuff. Halleluiah! I was so happy for him and proud of him I could hardly contain myself. He worked ridiculously hard on organizing everything he wanted to say and do while working a full-time job and being a husband and father. Eventually I got the call and he told me the filming date. I was excited and scared. I was never a good public speaker (not that I had to talk in this) and I desperately did not want to let him down (since I was the only other person that knew the system now).

The morning of the video shoot was an early one and we worked ALL day. I was very sore and exhausted when we left - being thrown around and beat up by a huge man for 8 hours will do that to you! But I still managed to drag myself out to a party after supper. When I arrived, I had trouble getting out of the car and found myself a little shocked and embarrassed, so I sucked it up and did my best to walk normally. As the evening progressed, my pain worsened (despite the booze) and I actually started worrying a little. My whole body felt like I'd been run over several times by a herd of buffalo, but my legs were on fire, especially my quads. Now keep in mind that I was in crazy good, strong shape at this point, it wasn't like I got off the couch and did this monumental workout cold. I quit drinking and left the party early very eager to crawl into bed and pray for a better morning.

No such luck. I slept terribly due to the pain and in the morning, I was greeted by visibly swollen and bruised thighs, knees crying out for ice packs and calves that were doing that little twitchy dance just before dropping into a brutal Charlie horse. WTF? As I hobbled to the kitchen for ice, I replayed the day before in my head and started piecing together the injuries. Most of the counter attacks/defense moves in his system required me to stun/surprise the attacker then sprint away to safety, not stand toe to toe with an aggressive male. Usually, I had been knocked down, so that initial launch up from the ground and furious first few steps til I was off camera had chewed up my legs something fierce. Once or twice or even a dozen times would have been fine, but we did it repeatedly for hours and hours. My adrenaline and excitement had dulled any foreboding warning bells the day of and now I was paying for it.... BIG TIME. Sitting and standing were the worst and I adopted a leaning, rolling method to help my incinerated muscles for about a week. Once recovered, we got bad news. The filming guys were giving Chris the run-around and a hard time. I don't know all the details but suffice it to say they were being arse-holes. He was so bummed out. Not only had he worked immensely hard preparing everything, but it also cost him a ton of money. We continued working out and perfecting the system and eventually he wanted to try again to make a video. Luckily, my brother, who is an artistic director in theatre was willing to help us out and also had access to filming equipment. So, we got ready for round two! We finished filming the second attempt and I was exhausted again, but not as sore this time (thankfully). He wasn't happy with the end result for several reasons even though it was much better than the first go-round and then life got in the way. He was dealing with a divorce and custody issues of his 2 small children and a career change and I went blind in one eye and got diagnosed with lupus and had new physical limitations and a messy breakup. Basically, shit happened. Following this cluster fuck, he eventually met someone new, settled down and started his new business and I met someone new and moved far away and we lost touch. He did contact me once when his ex-wife started dating someone who I used to party with many moons ago and we had a nice talk and catch up session. I do miss him and our friendship terribly and he was a huge part of my life for 7 years, but it seems like our lives drifted apart due to, well, life! I can only hope that he continued on with his dream because his ideas have the potential to help millions and if there was anyone who ever deserved to succeed it is him. It just goes to show that you never really know the impact you have in other people's lives and I'm forever grateful for the time he was in mine. He is a one in a million type of guy who brought out the best in me and made me believe in myself.

Thanks buddy!

PS if you need a glowing reference letter for any future job, feel free to show them this! :)

Helicopter

Driving home after a long day at work I came face to face with a scene straight out of TV. I lived out of town and usually my drive home got quieter as I left the city, but not today. My road was blocked by 2 police cars with lights flashing and several officers standing there. There was a ton of emergency vehicles about a mile beyond them. An officer approached my car and told me I'd have to turn around. I explained that my house was just in front of the commotion and I was concerned for my dogs because of all the chaos. He got on his radio then told me I could go ahead as long as I promised to go slow, stay out of everyone's way and make sure I pulled my car on my lawn if I couldn't access my driveway. I agreed, he moved his cruiser and I drove home. Luckily, I was able to squeak in the driveway (I had a pretty steep ditch out front that I was hoping not to have to attempt to drive through). My dogs were nutty and visibly relieved to have me home (Have you SEEN/HEARD what's going on out there mom????). I got them settled and quickly called my neighbour to see if he knew anything.

Very sadly, he relayed the terrible story to me. There was a horse stable on the property behind ours with a very long driveway out to our road. Tragically, a young teenage girl was riding a horse who spooked on her. He bolted down the driveway at full speed and she was unable to stop him. He broke right through the gate onto the road and smack into an SUV going about 90km/hr. The girl, the driver and the passenger were all injured but alive. Sadly, the horse was severely injured but alive and the authorities shot him to end his agony. I was dumbfounded, but before I could even reply, a huge noise started shaking the house and the dogs proceeded to lose their minds. I'd never heard anything like it. It took me a few seconds to realize that it was a helicopter - landing in my front yard! I shit you not, it landed directly in front of my house on the road. The EMS workers were ready and loaded 2 of the victims. Only a few minutes later another one landed for the 3rd victim. Not wanting to be a "looky-loo" and trivialize this terrible tragedy I stayed inside.

The police stayed for about an hour afterwards. The poor horse was picked up with a tractor and brought back to the farm to be buried. Eventually my neighbour and I came out and just kind of stared at each other open mouthed and stammering. The silence after something so chaotic laid on us like a heavy wet blanket. Even the dogs were solemn and quiet, like they knew what had just happened.

Definitely not an upbeat story, but a unique one I sincerely hope to never experience again.

Sweeping

Of all the jobs or job offers I've had, this is definitely the strangest. In my mid 20's I was on a mission for an interesting, fulfilling job. I, once again, was getting bored and wanted to find something with some pizzazz. I interviewed at a couple specialty clinics, looked into a wildlife rabies team and a few other places that fell outside the norm. But by far, the most interesting one was an outdoor safari park.

I was really excited to interview there because I had done a lot of research on them and had discovered they had a couple of captive breeding programs to help endangered species. I was on board and ready to nail this. Besides my RVT background, medical knowledge, animal experience and excitement, I was sincerely passionate about contributing to a monumentally important project like saving an endangered species. Let's do this.

When I met the man who was interviewing me, all I noticed was how tired he was. He was a nice guy but seemed like he'd just run a marathon. I took this as my cue to up my enthusiasm to make him feel like I'd really be a benefit there and take some of his workload off him. We talked for a while and then he asked me what position I was shooting for. When I explained that I'd like to get into, he looked at me really strangely and said he was only interviewing for animal husbandry jobs. I jumped in and said I was well aware that I'd have to start at the bottom and work my way up, but that I would like to start at the bottom of the area I wanted to climb the ladder in, not just a random job. He sighed and leaned back in his chair and told me that there was a waiting list of years full of people with more letters after their names than in their names for those positions. Vets, doctors, med students, researchers, etc. I was bummed.

He reread my application and told me that he liked me, that he thought I was over qualified for what he had to offer but that he wanted me on his team. I was disappointed with the breeding program news but interested in what he had to say.

"I could start you off at minimum wage as a monkey sweeper."

Excuse me what???? I was confused but thought it was his tired attempt at a joke. Nope. Turns out that staff are posted at the gates between the outdoor enclosures to sweep monkeys off the visitor's cars before they drive through to the predator enclosures! I laughed my ass off! He smiled and said that was all he had. I politely declined, shook his hand and left - laughing all the way to my car.

I was definitely disappointed, but I couldn't stop smiling. I mean really, if I gave you a week to come up with the most obscure job you could think of, would monkey sweeping even enter your brain???

Poop

I have heard many times from many different people that getting pooped on by a bird is supposed to bring good luck. I cannot vouch for any of these people's state of intoxication at the time that they offered said wisdom. Regardless, I should be one lucky S.O.B. because I have been the recipient of this "gift" 3 times. On top of that, all 3 times were at one of my favorite places in the world - The Molson Amphitheatre (now called the Budweiser Stage). It is hands down, the world's best place to go to a concert. Especially a loud concert. For those that don't know it (shame on you) it is on the edge of the water in Toronto, Ontario and seats about 16,000 people. It has a partial roof which covers about 2/3 of the crowd and the back 1/3 is open to the elements. I'm no expert sound tech but as a multiple repeat customer, I can tell you that it's awesome. Having no walls and no obstacles the sound is crystal clear, with no reverb, feedback, static or echo. I can't even count the number of shows I've seen there. I've also been to countless shows at enclosed venues and there's just no comparison.

One particular show strikes me as I write this. More years ago, than I care to count, I went to a Metallica concert at a huge enclosed arena in Toronto (which shall remain nameless). I was really excited because I'd always wanted to see them. NO FAULT of the band - I'm pretty sure they did a hell of a job - but 3 songs into their set, we were so disappointed because of the ridiculous amount of echo and feedback. We were actually late cheering, because the song kept going about 10 seconds after they were done! About 5 songs into their set, we could barely see them anymore because of all the pyrotechnic smoke (and cigarette and weed smoke). The smoke had nowhere to go and was slowly filling up the stadium. It was a real let down (again, not the band's fault). I share this negative experience not to trash the other venue, but only to express the awesomeness of Molson.

That said, I must air my beef about the wildlife inhabiting Molson. The first and third time I was used as a bathroom, it was from seagulls. Not pleasant. First time was on my head (thankfully I wear a hat, but still gross). Third time was on my neck and shoulder (still warm too) which I have yet to figure out his flight path to achieve that trajectory. But #2 was a doozy. My friend and I were sitting on the lawn section waiting for the show to start and I felt someone tap me on the leg several times, so I turned to talk to them. I didn't know them, but concerts can be friendly places, so I turned with a smile. The lady had her back to me, so I was confused for a moment.... until I realized my leg was warm. I looked down to find 3 large chunks of Canada goose shit resting happily on my leg, soaking into my jeans. (FYI Canada geese shit like cats in formed, tootsie roll type logs, not the runny white stuff like most birds). The group of people around me busted up with laughter and lots of advice.

Here are my issues with all the proceeding events:

1. I am 5'2". Both times I was standing up (Poop #1 and #3) I was surrounded by people easily a full foot taller than me that would have logically been better and easier targets.
2. Why the hell would any wild bird want to be anywhere near such a noisy, chaotic event?
3. There was 15999 other f'n people there! Seriously, you couldn't pick someone else for once??

Poop aside, I will forever be a Molson Amphitheatre customer. If only I could convince them to drop the price of beer. $15/can seems steep especially since there's such a high risk of it being pooped on!

Rock Path

I got my dream job. I got it! After years of passing the idea off because it was unlikely to happen and the idea of it was not very realistic or practical, it actually happened. Believe it or not, I actually have my blindness to thank for it too. After going blind in my right eye, fighting through all the chaos and misdiagnosis, losing my job (because I was now a "liability"), losing my boyfriend (because it was too much for HIM to handle...WTF?) and readjusting to my vision issues, I had one of those "a-ha" moments. Insert corny cliché here - Life's too short, etc. I had lost everything (I thought) and I wasn't going to waste anymore time. I was on the hunt for my dream job. Through some college connections and following up some pretty vague leads, I landed an interview at a mid-sized Standardbred horse breeding farm. I had no interest in the racing, but to be around horses all day, every day and be able to deliver the foals was something I knew I'd both excel at and enjoy, and I finally realized that it was no longer about the paycheck for me, I needed to enjoy life more.

I went to that interview like a woman possessed. There was no way in hell that I was letting this slip by. The owners lived on the property and I ended up in their kitchen for 3 hours, then took a property tour. The place was like something out of a movie. They kept between 50-80 horses, depending on the time of year and had about 100 acres (50-theirs, 50-rented). I was floating on air. Waiting for the call was torture, but eventually it came. Yes!

I had been around horses for decades and had delivered tons of calves, pigs, dogs, cats, sheep and I really enjoy being outside and doing physical labour, so I was very comfortable in my ability to excel at this job. The only intimidating part was the shear expense of some of the animals. There were 2 different mares on the property that were worth a million a piece and many others in the hundreds of thousands. In my opinion, a horse is a horse and a free one can break their leg the same as one worth a few bucks. But being responsible for these animals did come with just a tad more stress. There was a very eclectic group of staff to keep things interesting too. I busted ass and was never happier. I worked tons of hours and during foaling season I worked midnights (a few stories from those times later). During midnight shifts, of course I was tired, but there was something very peaceful about being in the barn at night, alone and connecting with these amazing animals. With the occasional burst of excitement when it was time to deliver a little munchkin. I was so addicted to it that I would push and push and push myself to ridiculous limits - during one foaling marathon, I worked 31 nights straight. Thirty-one. Eventually, my body had enough and started to shut down. There was one morning coming off work that I parked in my driveway, hobbled over towards the house, collapsed and literally crawled up my steps and passed out on my kitchen floor. I had to face facts that something was wrong. I had ignored my body's signals for too long and I was scared of what the next development would be.

Thankfully, one of my bosses was a doctor and held a very high standing in the local hospitals and was able to help me out with some appointments and diagnostics. I was also still under the care of several doctors since my blindness/possible MS diagnosis. After some forced time off and lots of appointments the final conclusion was lupus. My heart was broken. I pushed harder and bargained with my body every day, begging it to stay strong so I could keep this job. No dice. At just under 3 years there, I had to leave for the safety of myself, the other staff and the horses. I was devastated and furious but at the rate my symptoms were overtaking me I had no choice. One of the worst symptoms I had was loss of strength and pretty severe pain in my hands, so to try and hang on to a crazy yearling stud colt became almost impossible and we had a couple dozen of them. Also, UV light worsens lupus symptoms so having an outdoor job was becoming very counter-productive. And the exhaustion - there really are no words to explain the intensity of the all-encompassing exhaustion. It's not like you're tired and need a nap, it's like you just ran a triathlon then spent 4 hours lifting weights at the gym, then stayed up partying for 48 hours. Every appendage on your body feels like it weighs 500 pounds.

After I left, I was in a very dark place and was feeling and dealing with so much rage I kind of zoned out for awhile. I went through the motions of daily life, but I wasn't really present. I desperately wanted to go back to the farm and visit but only managed to do it once because it was just so fucking painful. When I did go back, I went out into a huge field with about 15 broodmares in it and found my girl - a stunningly beautiful and powerful mare named Glacier. She had been my favorite since day one. She was definitely used to me loving her up but that day when I walked to her, she knew something was different. She was one of the top-ranking mares in the herd and she made short work of getting the rest of them to back off, then she stood her ground under this huge, knarly old tree and I collapsed onto her, burying my face into her neck and hugging her while I sobbed uncontrollably. I felt so betrayed by my body, so unsafe and so alone. But holding her - I knew I was safe with her and she made me feel grounded and a whole lot stronger. She never flinched, never moved a muscle. She just stood there for the longest time, letting me indulge in her scent, feel her solid and supportive muscles and deep rhythmic breathing and soak her beautiful copper coat with tears. When I finally came up for air, she stayed with me. When I walked the 1/2 mile back to the truck, she (and some of the others) walked back with me. Sure, some of them came in hopes of grain but not Glacier. I climbed the gate, hugged her again, kissed her many times and thanked her from the depths of my soul. With one final kiss on the nose, I choked out my goodbye and left. When I looked back in the rear-view mirror, she was still standing there.

Thank you, Glacier.

Rock Path Stories

There were a few more noteworthy stories that came out of my time at the horse barn;

1. While doing evening chores in the summer, I met something that stopped me in my tracks. I was going through the motions, visiting and feeding all the barns. Then I hopped in the old truck and headed out to the fields were the broodmares were to check on everyone and top up water tanks. Everything was fine, and I was in a great mood, thoroughly loving life, the horses and my job. I swear there might as well have been birds flitting around my head singing. The weather was beautiful, the day had gone well, and I was almost done for the day. I climbed up the 4 ft high gate, swung my leg over and just before I dropped down on the other side I froze. Holy shit! That was a huge flippin' snake! Now, don't get me wrong, I love snakes. I think they are amazingly cool and interesting creatures, but this guy was really big, and I came within about 2 ft of stepping directly on him - which I'm sure he would not have appreciated! I sat there for several minutes just looking at him. He didn't seem bothered at all by my presence and just laid there sunbathing in the worn-down grass. All the grass in the paddock was either chewed down by the horses or about 3 ft tall, so this spot by the gate must have been prime real estate and he was in no hurry to move. I wish that I had a camera (or a cell phone with a camera) at the time because I would have loved to take pictures of him. First off to warn the other staff and second to find out what he was. I don't know much about snakes, but he definitely did not look like any of the native species that I knew about. He was about 4 ft long, as big around as a pop can and a strange beige/orange colour with some bumps on his head. I looked on the internet later but never found anything that matched. My best guess was that someone had an exotic pet that they let loose or he was some

genetic abnormality of a native snake. Either way, I was super grateful he didn't bite me! Eventually he moved off into the tall grass and none of us ever saw him again. The other staff teased me about telling a fish story, thinking he was only a 6-inch-long garter snake, but the image of that big dude is still sharp in my brain even all these years later. I was always a lot more careful walking through the tall grass after that and tried to keep my Snow-White fairy tale singing to a minimum!

2.   Another staff member and I had gone out to the rental fields at the far end of the property one ridiculously cold winter morning to bring in a small group of mares. It was the kind of cold that freezes your nostril hair and can freeze a cup of water thrown in the air before it lands. We had to walk because the snow was too deep for the truck. On the way up, we periodically swung gates and locked them to make a safe path for the horses to walk freely back to the barn - we sure as hell weren't going to walk back and forth to bring them all in separately in thigh deep snow. Also, once they tramped down the snow it would be way easier for us. There was 8 of them and they were very happy to see us. However, they were not too happy when we jammed our freezing cold hands into their nice toasty warm armpits! What happened next defies all explanation. There literally are no words I can use to do justice to what we saw. The mares were very spirited, and they took off through the snow en masse, side by side, snorting. The thundering of their hooves was intense and shook the ground under our feet. The sun was in front of them, full force, not a cloud in the sky. They kicked up immense plumes of snow that twinkled and sparkled in the sun. It was the most beautiful sight I had ever seen. We stood there for about 2 minutes completely awestruck. It was like something out of a dream. I looked at her, she looked at me and we walked back to the barn in silence. Once we got there the ethereal beings had turned back into horses and were staring at us, impatient for

breakfast. We really didn't talk about it afterwards because we didn't know how to put it in words, just like I'm having trouble doing now. It was a beautiful sight like nothing else I've ever witnessed before or since.

3.   As I said before, we worked with a lot of stud colts who were unpredictable at best. We had handled them daily since infancy, so they were used to us and the rules of the barn, but were still very large, very fiery, VERY hormonal boys. The fillies were kept in a totally separate wing of the main barn and we always worked with them after the boys, so as not to bring any girly aromas over to the frat house. There was however, one other problem. Two of the top-ranking boys.... well...."liked" me when it was my time of the month. One was worse than the other, but both became quite comical (when in their stalls) and quite dangerous (when out of their stalls) around me. All I had to do was walk in the barn and they would start calling to me, pacing their stalls, kicking the walls, snorting and becoming very agitated. There were other women in the barn, but it appeared that I was the only one whose hormones crossed the species barrier! You can't even imagine how much teasing I put up with. If either of those colts even farted, the staff would say things like, "Oh no, better get Stacy some chocolate and a Midol!" There was one scary time where I was working with one of them (because my period had not started yet) and he was crazy affectionate and nuzzling me and chuffing to me and leaning on me (kind of like a drunk guy in a bar). I was correcting him but eventually decided to put him back in his stall for safety. When I turned, he went straight up and tried to mount me! Thankfully, his chest knocked me down and out of the way. I was back on my feet with lightning speed and he was back in his stall even faster. Funniest thing was though that he was accurate - my period started that night! I often wondered if there was any way to get those 2 a job helping women with fertility issues!

Norman Or'deurves

One night while working the midnight shift at the horse farm, I had an unforgettable experience that I shared with our barn cat Norman.

I was alone on a 50-acre farm. It was winter, and my job was to deliver the foals of these prize racehorses. As any midwife will tell you, most births happen at night and horses are no different. Their babies also get a kick out of stressing everyone out at 3 in the friggin' morning!

Anyways, we had a birth, which is amazing, adrenaline pumping and exhausting (but amazing.... did I mention that??) Mom and baby were doing great, so I was able to get tidying up and preparing for our next bundle of joy. After inspecting the afterbirth, it was customary to bring it outside to the manure pile and bury it, so it can decompose. So off I go with my wheelbarrow of goodies and my trusty right-hand-man Norman trotting along beside me through the dark arena towards the back door.

Normally, stepping out on a perfectly cold, calm, quiet night like that would be an enjoyable breath of fresh air after working up a sweat from being armpit deep inside a horse......but not tonight. Instantly the hair on the back of my neck stood up and it wasn't from the cold. I couldn't hear or see anything but even Norman stopped and sniffed the air. I stood there for a minute, told myself I was being silly (mistake) and pressed on down the driveway (bigger mistake). I got about 20 feet when I stopped dead in my tracks - there was eye shine 20 feet away. Not a huge animal, but definitely bigger than a racoon or possum. I stared at it a few seconds, neither of us moving until something else caught my eye. You guessed it - more eye shine. This time directly in front of me, only about 10 feet away. I heard a twig snap behind me and my "stealth mode" was abruptly replaced with "get me the hell out of here mode"! I dropped the wheelbarrow and as I spun around, I saw 1/2 dozen more eye shines to the left and further back. In my entire life I have never moved as fast as I did in those next few seconds (if I even took that long)

About halfway back to the barn I saw good ol' Norman frozen in full kitty defence mode and as I sprinted by him I reached down and grabbed the poor guy by his hind leg/butt/tail region (thankfully I had my heavy winter barn coat on as he less than pleased about my choice of holds and he hung on for dear life with all of his claws). We got in the barn and closed the 20x20 foot sliding door in a heartbeat with the strength of 10 men (any of you who have had to heave one of those heavy buggers in the winter, with snow drifts know that's no easy feat). Norman and I ran into the back office/lunch room, slammed the door and raced to look out the window to try and see our would-be attackers. What I saw was a large pack of coyotes knock over my wheelbarrow and take off with their prize. Within a minute of their departure, the night exploded with their songs and yips of excitement, which, up until that night, I had always enjoyed hearing!

You know, I'm a reasonable person. They have to eat - not my choice for a delicacy - but couldn't we have figured out some sort of drive-thru window situation??

Moral of the story: ALWAYS trust your gut. Especially if your only back up is a 10-pound barn cat!

Norman 2

On a different midnight shift at the horse barn I had another situation happen involving good ol' Norman. It was winter, it was the middle of the night and I had just arrived to start my shift. The place was dark, and I was attempting to pull open the heavy barn door that had a fair-sized snow drift in front of it with my arms full of stuff. I got it open a crack, just wide enough to squeeze through, so I pushed my lunch box and stuff through first and then wiggled the rest of me in. In the midst of trying not to wipe out I was accosted by Norman, who kept getting under foot. I didn't want to hurt him, but I couldn't see a thing, the barn was even darker than outside, so I kept pushing him away with my foot and once with my hand. He was pretty determined, but not as determined as I was to find the damn light switch! I felt my way along the wall and flipped on the light. I turned around to give Norman shit for being such a pain and boy was I surprised. It wasn't Norman. There was a flippin' possum rooting around my lunch box! I let out a squeal and it hissed at me and slowly plodded out into the indoor arena. I was definitely awake for my shift now. How I didn't get bitten is beyond me. I touched him half a dozen times with my foot and once with my hand and he never made a sound. To say I was lucky was an understatement. The real Norman sauntered out to greet me about 20 minutes later wondering what all the fuss was about.

Most nights, I tried to keep everything quiet and as dark as possible for the horse's comfort, but that night ALL the lights were on! I wasn't about to tempt fate for the 7th time in a row!

Camel

So, every vet clinic has it's share of eccentric clients and there's one that really sticks out for me. The lady was incredibly nice, sweet and loving and crazy smart. She and her husband were both university professors. I never dealt with him but saw her regularly because she was always calling or coming in for something for her 100 plus animals! Now, to be clear, she was not a hoarder and her pets were all well taken care of and she had a huge acreage with several barns. How she afforded to take care of them all was beyond me. Every animal was vaccinated, neutered and provided with any emergency treatment needed. She had everything - dogs, cats, rabbits, goats, sheep, cattle, horses, pigs, etc - all of which were rescued. But my favorite by far were her two camels that were rescued from a circus. She had a male and a female. The female was tame, but the big male was a little rougher around the edges.... unless he liked you. I was lucky enough to have made the cut and I was able to scratch and pet him whereas my male boss definitely did not! So once a year when we went to do a farm call and examine/vaccinate all the critters, he was my responsibility. I'd never seen a camel up close before and I was blown away by his size - he was HUGE. The lady had customized 1/2 of one barn for him so he'd be comfortable.

When it was his turn, the lady would get a bucket of treats for him and open a small man door and he'd put his head out and happily munch away (his body wouldn't fit out). After he'd checked thoroughly to make sure there was no men around and had received enough initial lovin' from the ladies. His head was 3/4 the length of my body, he smelled terrible and he drooled continuously but he was so cool! He used to make this weird rumbly, purring, thundery sound when he was happy that was like nothing I'd ever heard before. As he ate, I would rub and scratch all over his neck and quickly vaccinate him before he even knew what had happened and then continue loving him up. Thankfully he always preferred the attention over trying to kill us over the tiny poke in the neck because I can only imagine the damage he was capable of inflicting.

Pit Bulls

Working at a humane society is both a blessing and a curse. You have to see firsthand how horribly cruel and evil people can be. It can easily make you full of rage/hate and fearful of civilization (ex. An 8-week-old kitten brought in because its skin was peeling off because a man had thrown it in a bucket of bleach to "teach his girlfriend a lesson". I euthanized it immediately to put an end to its unexplainable torturous suffering.) But then there are also many times where you are part of an incredibly good thing that makes your heart pull a Grinch and swell up 10 times its normal size. (ex. adoptions, shutting down puppy mills, getting helpless animals out of horrific hoarding situations, seeing a community band together and help against a few rotten apples).

Unfortunately, this story does not have a happy ending, but the message is of utmost importance and needs to be shared to spread awareness. It deals with a topic that is close to my heart, ENDING DOG FIGHTING. How anyone could engage in this activity is beyond all reason and human decency. It is far more prevalent than the general public realizes and needs to end NOW. I could write a whole book on this topic, I'm so passionate about it but I'm going to focus on one story that I had firsthand experience with. First though, I'd encourage you to read up on the dog fighting catastrophe online and help in any way you can. I also want to state a few facts:

1. Pitbulls ARE NOT bad dogs and should never be judged by the actions of the douchebags who make them fight.
2. Dogs do not naturally fight to the death/serious grievous injuries over nothing.
3. Dog fighting a-holes should all give their dogs to loving homes and start betting on MMA fights. At least those participants are there by choice.

Anyways, I was head of the Animal Health Department and I got an upsetting call from our Cruelty Investigations Officer one beautiful summer day. She was bringing me in a dog with bad injuries she had seized from a dog fighting group. She needed the Animal Care Attendants to set up an isolated run for him and needed me ready to check him out and help him. When she arrived, my heart broke. She lifted him on the exam table and he limply wagged his tail and licked my hand. I shoved down all my tears and got to work. You couldn't even tell what colour he was because of all the dried blood and fresh blood. I cleaned all the blood off him gently and bandaged the most severe injuries. He never offered to bite. He never moved. He never growled. I can't even imagine how much pain he was in. We then sent him off to the local vet for some sutures and legal documentation. He came back in about an hour and we set him up in his kennel. Unfortunately, because of the waste-of-skin owners, he had massive dog aggression, so we had to keep him sedated during his stay for his benefit and peace of mind. Hard to heal when you are on high alert and stressed out. We also had to padlock his kennel door - for safety, for legality and accountability. There were only 2 keys, one for me and one for the Officer.

His name was Tyson (real original to name a fighting dog after Mike Tyson. Did you use all 3 of your brain cells to come up with that one boys???). Tyson and I became REALLY close over the next several weeks. I was his caregiver, his nurse, his friend and his official belly rubber, nose kisser and hand feeder. His physical wounds healed nicely but his emotional ones will probably never completely heal. During the time he was with us, the staff was under constant attack from the gang that owned him. They came to the shelter, they called all the time. They threatened, they peacocked, they made us scared to go outside or drive home at night. Have I mentioned that we need to get tougher laws for these losers? One of them actually told me that he was going to follow me home. The police said there was nothing they could do because the roads are public and there was no direct threat after the "follow you home" part. Well I don't think he was coming to swap recipes or paint my toenails!

Anyways, the real heartbreak came when the case was thrown out of court because of a stupid clerical error on some paperwork. Really judge?? Devastatingly, we had to release him back to them. We were so disgusted and depressed. The entire staff was mortified. The police showed up at the shelter to supervise the event. The scumbags showed up, in a limo. Laughing. They made a big production and mockery of it. I was physically ill and shaking with rage. Why the hell did this happen? How the hell can those demons look in that sweet dogs' eyes and do what they do? Worst of all, how can that poor dog wag his tail when he saw them? I cried like I never cried before. I'm crying right now as I write this and remember that sweet dog.

I am begging you. Please do your part to end dog fighting. There are many ways you can help. You can volunteer your time at a shelter, donate funds to shelters and rescue groups, lobby politicians and government to toughen up the current laws so there are actually consequences for animal abuse, just be aware and report ANY suspicious activity to the police.

Trainer

I always wear a baseball hat. Anyone who does likewise, knows about that damn little button right on the top. If I'm going to bump my head, it always seems to be right on the button - which of course "up's" the ouch factor. Well, one day, I took the ouch factor way up and out of the stratosphere.

While working in the dairy barn, doing morning chores after milking (cows were all outside, I was prepping an empty barn). I was zoned out with repetitiveness and routine. I was finished chopping straw for bedding and now I was spreading it out and fluffing it up for my girls. Moving from stall to stall, I got into an unconscious rhythm, so when I heard a loud bang it startled me, and I spun around to see what it was. Then I felt like someone hit me on the head with a baseball bat and everything went dark.

You see, I'm short, only 5'2" and the electric trainers in a dairy barn (a small thin piece of metal that hangs down over the cow to give her a zap if she hunches up too much to poop, thereby keeping her bedding clean and dry) generally hang around that height. As I spun and straightened, I made direct contact with the electric trainer and the little metal button on the top of my hat which of course was connected to my skull! I must have dropped like a bag of hammers. When I came to, I had a hell of a headache and a red welt on my scalp. I figured I'd been out about 5 minutes (thankfully, it was all fresh, soft bedding I landed in)

Now, embarrassingly, I have been zapped before by electric fences and once by a prod - courtesy of the arse-holes I used to work with (thanks guys). I'm pretty sure this incident wouldn't have been so bad if it hadn't connected with that damn little button, but I'm sure not going to test the theory!

Therapy Animals

I have had the opportunity to work with various animals, enriching the lives of seniors through St John's Ambulance and privately. These are some of the best stories.

1. JACK

I started with my awesome dog Jack, my friend Kari and her amazing dog Mr Moo (who would eventually join my herd). We did all the testing, passed with flying colours and were excited to start our visits.

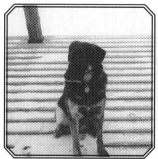
Jack

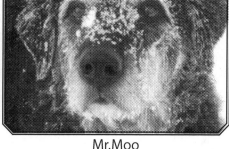
Mr.Moo

We were assigned to a nursing home and upon arrival, we were each sent in different directions. They were both large dogs (Jack - 90lbs, Mr Moo - 100lbs) and it was wonderful to see the looks on the male residents faces. You see, most of the visiting dogs were small/toy sized dogs, so the men were excited to see some big old boys. One man could barely contain himself and was scooting along in his walker all hunched over and hollering at me. He was so worried he was going to miss seeing Jack! I doubled my pace, concerned the old guy might wipe out. When we met up, he was winded but happy and he sat down on his walker. He started roughly petting Jack's head with his knarled old hands while he told me all about the dogs he'd had as a young man. You don't need a college degree to see the ridiculously huge benefit he was experiencing. He was laughing, smiling, telling stories and even straightened up noticeably. He told me about his friend a few doors down that was bedridden that I just HAD to go see next. I said sure and as we started out, he stopped me and asked if Jack could shake a paw. You know how sometimes time goes in slow motion and you still can't catch an impending disaster?? As he said the words "shake a paw" while extending his hand, I dropped to my knees and attempted (unsuccessfully) to block the large black paw hurtling towards the man. Too late. Jack landed his paw on the old man with laser accuracy and the enthusiastic power of a large young dog......and the old man went down! To the floor! I desperately tried to help him up while trying to shield him from the barrage of sloppy dog kisses raining down around him, while simultaneously wondering if I was going to jail. The man was laughing his ass off and had tears streaming from his eyes. A nurse rushed over, I put Jack in a down, stay and we lifted the man up. My eyes were wide, I was repeatedly apologizing, and I was 10 shades of red. Nice impression to make on my maiden voyage. The nurse was glaring at me, Jack's tail was wagging 100km/hr and the man was still smiling. He reached out, grabbed my hand in both of his, looked me right in the eyes and said the most sincere "thank you" I'd ever heard in my life. He said that was the most excitement he'd had in years! Due to his glowing report we weren't black listed or arrested, but I did learn a valuable lesson: A hunched over 90-year-old, top heavy man sitting on an unstable walker is no match for a 90lb exuberant dog with large paws who shook them like a frat boy slamming down an empty beer mug on a bar!

PS I started working on "gentle shake" that very night with Jack!

2. STINKY PETE

Through one of the vet clinics I worked at, I met a lady who worked at a nursing home. We got to talking and I mentioned how I used to bring my dog to a seniors home for visits (omitting the above story of course!) She said they had lots of dogs, but that many residents were requesting a cat visit. Now, due to the inherent nature of cats, they aren't exactly the perfect choice for visitation to a senior's home. Nails, teeth, low annoyance threshold, dislike of car rides, dislike of new surroundings, dislike of new people, etc, etc. I thought for only a second and then proceeded to volunteer myself and tell her all about my cat Stinky Pete. He was a great big, fluffy, sweet heart who'd had his head crushed in a sliding glass door as a kitten with his previous owner. He was surrendered to our clinic a few years later because the owner had become a hoarder and was ordered to give up a dozen cats. Pete was blind in one eye (from the accident) but unbelievably sweet so I took him home hoping he'd mellow out my little tiny firecracker kitty, Evil. His original name was Precious, I switched it to Pete and then it quickly became Stinky Pete due to his gas issues. Anyways, maybe he had brain damage from his head injury or maybe he was just mind-blowingly sweet, but I thought if ANY cat had a chance at therapy work, it was him! The lady was so ecstatic. We booked him in the very next week.

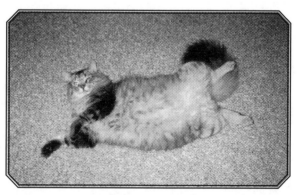

Sweet Stinky Pete

He got quite a turnout, almost 20 resident ladies had made the trip to the common room and had set up in a large circle. I figured there was really not much I could do except open the crate door and hope for the best. I was stunned at what he did. That amazing cat sauntered around the circle like he owned the place, letting everyone pet him and stopping a few times to lay down and offer his belly for a rub! Most dogs wouldn't handle a strange situation with that many new people that well! Just another day at the office for good ol' Pete. We went back several more times with the same results - happy cat, happy residents, happy staff, happy me. One day I went back the co-ordinator asked if I'd be willing to take him to the dementia floor. I had some experience with my own grandmother on a dementia/Alzheimer's ward, so I had at least some idea what to expect. My only concern was for Pete's safety as sometimes the patients can lash out. The co-ordinator assured me that the "prone to violence" residents were not allowed to attend and that there would be plenty of staff on hand this time to help. When I got up there, there was only 8 residents and 6 staff, so I felt pretty good. I let Pete out and he proceeded to be his regular charming self. He wasn't fazed by the unpredictable behaviour or noise.

A teeny tiny woman wheeled up beside me and asked, "What's his name dear?" in a sweet little pixie voice. "Pete" I proudly answered. "Oh, that's lovely dear!" About 10 seconds later she tapped me on the arm "What's his name dear?" "Pete" I said, thinking she hadn't heard me the first time. "Oh, that's lovely dear!" This continued for the remainder of the visit. The next time I went back the tiny lady was front and centre with the look of a little kid at Christmas. My heart broke for her. I really hoped that Pete would spend some extra time with her. Her line of repetitive questioning began immediately. About halfway through the hour, I looked to the nurses for help. They just smiled and said to ignore her because it would never stop. I have the utmost respect for nurses, but it just didn't sit right with me to ignore her, so I tried another tactic to still engage with her while trying to keep things fun and light.

"What's his name dear?"

"Ozzy Osbourne!"

"Oh, that's lovely dear!"

"What's his name dear?"

"Magnum P.I.!"

"Oh, that 's lovely dear!"

"What's his name dear?"

"Brian Bosworth!"

"Oh, that's lovely dear!"

This went on and on and on. I used every name I could think of and even used the internet to search interesting names before I went on my visits. It made the repetition far more tolerable and allowed her to stay involved and curious and feel heard, even if she forgot 2 seconds later!

3. Summertime Bob

While working at the dairy barn after graduating, I was lucky enough to be in charge of our nursery of calves. It was very slobbery work, but I loved those little guys. There was one bull calf in particular that I fell for. He had a dog-like personality and was quite comical. My boss didn't like me naming the bull calves because he knew how upset I got when they had to be shipped. For whatever reason, I started calling this little fart Bob (just between me and him). I was busted only a few days later when one of the guys overheard me. Only he heard "Summertime Bob" when I had said, "Geez, take some more time Bob!" referring to his slow milk intake (he liked to play in his milk bucket). I was teased about his dorky name (even though that wasn't his name).

Later that week, my boss was talking to friends of his while I finished up chores and I heard something about animal visits to seniors. I wasn't eavesdropping, but in a large open barn full of cows, machinery and huge fans, they had to talk pretty loudly. I asked what was going on and he said a local senior's home was asking around about getting some small farm animals to visit since most of the residents were from farms and were going stir crazy in their new accommodations. Without even thinking, I blurted out, "I'll take Bob!". The men looked at me strangely and shook their heads. "You can't take fucking cattle into an old folks' home!". Keep in mind that I was in my early 20's and full of piss and vinegar and NO ONE was gunna tell me what I could or couldn't do (just ask my parents, hee hee!). I'm sure they have a courtyard or something, we can make it work". I badgered them for a while more and then the man finally caved and said, "Ok, ok I'll call them". Needless, to say, a few days later I came in on my coveted day off to give Bob a bath and brush and loaded him in the truck (with help, he was a big bugger now). I brought along a student we had and off we went.

The reception was unbelievable! There must have been 50 people out on the lawn waiting for us. I opened up the truck and Bob launched out sideways and snorting. Hmmmmm....perhaps this wouldn't go as smoothly as Pete's visits......

Bob was not fond of being led around by the halter, so I let him have some freedom and he ended up voluntarily heading over to the people. The impact that dorky little calf had was incredible. The men especially started talking about "back in their day" and the herds they had and bloodlines, etc. I even heard a couple times something like, "I didn't know you had cattle, we should have a coffee and compare notes one day" By the end of our time there, I was soaked with sweat, I'd been pooped on and my hands were bleeding from the rope, but I felt so good about brightening everyone's day and potentially bringing a few people closer together, I didn't even care. We loaded him up on the trailer with remarkable ease. I think he was tired too from all his bucking bronco moves and that one time he tried to climb a tree…. seriously.

Thanks Bob, you were a special little dude!

Sabre-tooth Hedgehog

While working at an exotic animal practice can be very interesting, it can also be very challenging. One such challenge almost got my ass fired.

So, let's set the scene. My awesome cat "Stinky Pete" had some kind of seizure/stroke episode late the night before (Sunday)at home and I had been up all-night tending to him and worrying. Monday mornings are always loony in animal clinics because lots of owners ignore their animals' health issues all weekend and then think it's an emergency Monday morning, so we get swamped. Admittedly, my head was not in the game as I could hear my own cat yowling in distress no matter where I went in the clinic. We could not figure out what was wrong with him after an exam, blood work, x-rays, so we had booked him an ultrasound that afternoon. All I had to do was tough it through another couple of hours. I could do it...........

My quirky boss decided to submerge me in as much work as possible - I'm pretty sure it was with good intention to distract me. Anyways, she was asking for help with ridiculous things that she could have handled herself easily or with the help of a kennel attendant. Instead of distracting me she was frustrating the hell out of me because I was crazy busy myself. So, she asks me to come hold a hedgehog for her in the exam room - WTF??? For those new to hedgehogs, they are tiny little prickly critters smaller than a guinea pig who roll up in a spiny ball when stressed/scared. There is nothing to restrain. Exactly what was I supposed to do that her own hand/the table/the owner's hand couldn't do? Was I supposed to magically get it to spread eagle on the exam table by singing it a lullaby? It's a 3oz rodent! (though I'm hiding it well now, I was pretty pissed off then....)

But she did sign my paychecks at the time so in I went, wearing my best happy face.

The father and young daughter looked rather confused that the Dr. had called in reinforcements. It' s not like we were wrestling down a 150-pound dog or something. I merely smiled and held out my hand for the varmint. They handed over the well-armoured ball and I proceeded to zone out. I wasn't listening to all the conversation in the exam room, all I could hear was my poor cat's suffering. It felt like I'd been in there forever, and then WHAMO!!

That little piece of shit bit right THROUGH my thumb! Right in the sensitive crevice at the side of my fingernail. Here is the play-by-play account as told to me by the other tech who was out in the hall.

mumble, mumble

Me: FUCK!!

BANG! Ting, ting, ting

Boss: STACY!!

girl crying

Then she saw me running out of the room headed for the back, dripping blood all over the hall.

As I'm trying to wash my thumb, the full impact of what just happened comes flooding over me with tsunami intensity. Oh shit. The other tech came back wide-eyed with her mouth literally open. Oh shit. The boss comes back totally stone faced. Oh, double shit. She stares at me for an eternity. Oh shit, I'm fired. She shakes her head slowly and says, "I never thought I'd say something like this, but you're damn lucky your cat is dying."

I was grateful that it appeared I still had a job, but I was confused. She continued, "I explained what is going on to the owner and he was sympathetic to your situation. He even said that he and his wife have both tossed the little bugger when it bites them!" The hedgehog was completely fine, and once he landed, he uncurled and started walking around the exam room. Damn effective armour!

Obviously, they were not charged for their appointment and they had a permanent discount on their account, but can you believe they actually came back with the same damn hedgehog a few months later???

Clearly, this story doesn't paint me in a very good light, but it was strictly circumstantial I swear. It was just too ridiculous not to include it and if I didn't, all the people who know the story would have given me a hard time for not putting it in!

PS For those of you wondering what the sound effects were, the BANG was when I tossed him into the venetian blinds and the ting, ting, ting was the sound his spikes made as he rolled down the metal slats!

Vaccinating Cattle

You know when you have one of those dumb-ass moments that happen and after you recover, you quickly glance around like, "did anyone see that?" and either hang your head in shame or quickly scoot away victorious because you weren't caught? Well I had an inescapable one......literally.

I went out on a farm call with my boss (vet) to a large beef operation for a day of vaccinating. Which is very different than vaccinating your dog or cat or even horse. Depending on the numbers you're dealing with, the cattle are either run through a squeeze chute in a single line or sometimes there's enough head gates to hold them in their pens. This farm had both, so the vet decided to go outside and run the chute with the larger part of the herd and I stayed in the barn to vaccinate the younger ones in the head gates. They were already caught and happily munching away on breakfast. Easy peasy. I loaded my multidose syringe (looks like a gun but holds many doses so you're not fiddle farting around with 100's of individual syringes). Beef cattle are tough and unlike small animal medicine (and human) you only change the needle every 4-5 animals. This speeds up the process and cuts down on cost and waste.

Off I go, walking behind these 800-1000 lb steers, giving each one a scratch and then a poke in the rump. 90% of them didn't even look back or react. Like I said, easy-peasy. I was more than 1/2 done when I heard a gate clang shut behind me. Ever aware of the danger of being trampled by one of these big fella's if they got loose, I spun around to check it out. Gasp! There before me was farmer Joe's son. All 6'6", 275lbs of solid muscle with a sideways grin that could make a nun go to confession! I'd never met him before but had heard he was cute - understatement of the year. As he got closer and I struggled to regain my composure, he says,

"Just thought you might need a hand with some of these bruisers."

"I'm ok but sure you can help, thanks." I stammered.

My eyes were glued on him, but I returned to my autopilot job as he filled a second syringe. Then I slammed the needle directly through my hand between my thumb and forefinger then into the steer. Yep. I just vaccinated myself for bovine viral diarrhea and skewered myself to a very large, very dirty animal (you flirt your way, I'll flirt mine!). I let out a yell and Mr. Hotty spun around with eyes wide and mouth open. I looked down at my hand and back at him a few times then yanked the needle/hand combo out of the steer and then proceeded to pull it gingerly out of my own hand. Eeeeewww. Once it was out, it was his turn to stammer, "you ok?" with a bit of a pale face. I was bleeding badly, so I gave him the gun and said, "oh yeah, I'm fine, but I better clean this up!" with an overcompensating happy face. "Could you finish this pen please?" "Uh yeah."

I ran out to the truck and berated myself for my stupidity as I washed and wrapped my hand as best I could. Then my boss came over, quite concerned and I relayed MOST of the story. We went back to our jobs and finished up (with my ever swelling, throbbing hand). Thankfully, we finished quickly, and I never looked directly at Mr. Hunky again.

Once we were in the truck, my boss started asking me more questions and eventually figured it out. You know, for such a nice guy he had a hell of a mean streak! He roared with laughter and teased me all the way back to the clinic, then ran in ahead of me to tell everyone else.

My hand hurt for about 2 weeks, but my pride was sore for A LOT longer!

Fish from Hell

This story is embarrassing for me too but also so strange I had to share it. Back in the day, I was dating a guy who had an unusual pet. He kept telling me he had this amazing fish that I just had to see. Now, I love all critters, but I was not too excited about a fish - it's a fish.... woohoo. Well, I was sadly mistaken in my gross underestimation of this beast.

The first time I went to his house, he was really pumped up to show me his aquariums and I was pretty into him and impressed by his passion for these animals (even though they weren't dogs or horses). He had planned out my meet and greet and started me at the least impressive and we worked our way up to the grand finale. I don't remember all the species he had, but there were several tanks and I "oohed and aahhed" at the appropriate times. He was very knowledgeable and obviously dedicated a large amount of time to their care. He even had a tank just for the "feeder fish" that fed his piranhas and his special boy. Then he started to look like a little kid at Christmas, so I knew it was time for the main event. It was really funny to me because he was this tough biker with lots of tats, piercings, leather, etc and he was almost bouncing up and down and clapping his hands!

As we headed upstairs to the main floor, he pushed ahead and told me to wait. He turned off the main lights and turned on the tank light (oooh suspense...). Then proud as a peacock, he said it was time. I took a deep breath, reminded myself that I really liked this guy and went in. I made it about 3 feet into the room and froze with my mouth open. In front of me was something out of a horror movie. In a six-foot-long tank was a fish taking up almost half of it. He was an eerie white colour and reminded me of a moray eel. All that was bad enough but when I entered the room, he stopped swimming at the corner of the tank and stared at me.... I shit you not. That bugger stared at me for several minutes! I stared back in awe. Finally, my boyfriend laughed and walked over to me breaking the hypnotizing glare of his pet demon. I was stunned, I had never been intimidated by a fish before! Suddenly, I had way more interest in this thing and was talking a mile a minute asking questions.

Here's what I found out. He had seen him in the tank of feeder fish at the pet store when he was the size of a goldfish and knew he was special (shouldn't have been in that tank) and bought him and gave him his own tank. He did his research and found out that he was a rare albino Arowana worth lots of money, so he kept him and learned how to care for him. Arowana's are carnivorous fish that are nicknamed "water monkeys" because they can leap 6 feet out of the water to catch prey. Eeeek. Adult males are dominant and aggressive (no doubt) and can grow to 3 feet long in captivity - check. My boyfriend learned the hard way that these fish also do not like vacuum cleaners because while using it one day the fish jumped out of the water directly at the machine. When he tried to pick it up to put it back in the water, it bit him - severely enough to leave a scar on his wrist. From then on, he had to leave a Plexiglas cover on the tank, secured by a half dozen bricks so the behemoth couldn't escape. He also made a custom Plexiglas shield that he could use to pin the fish to 1/3 of the tank so he could safely clean it without being attacked.

We dated for about a year and a half and I swear that friggin' fish hated me right up until the very end. EVERY time I came in the house, he would stop swimming and glare at me for ridiculously long periods of time and sometimes even aggressively slap the water in my general direction! He never did that to my boyfriend or his 10-year-old daughter - just me. They thought it was quite funny. I thought it was creepy as hell. That thing gave me the heebie-jeebies because it was THINKING. It would methodically check the tank corners and top with little bumps, come back and stare at me, go chew up a terrified goldfish, come back and stare at me. Shudder. I know it sounds crazy, but I swear it's true! I fully admit that I was (and still am) terrified of a fish - albeit a huge, nightmarish, wanted to chew on my throat with its big teeth fish. I begged him to put a sheet over it when I was there, but he just laughed and said he'd eventually get used to me. Ya, get used to me or find a way out and bite my toe off! By the way, did I mention that they are capable of breathing air for short periods of time???? Creepy, creepy, creepy!!

"It"

Since my early teens, I have been on a never-ending quest for "more". Not for anything materialistic or money - just more out of life. It only worsened as I grew older. I could have a great job, nice place to live, active social life, my health, a reliable vehicle - basically everything I needed. I beat myself up a lot, thinking I was just greedy (and worse terms), but deep in my gut I knew there was "something" out there. I could play nice for a while, but it always came back, usually with more intensity each time. I was like a dog who knew he wasn't supposed to dig up the back yard, but after months of being good, he is overtaken by the overwhelming urge to search for something, some surprise, some unknown thing, "it". It drives me nuts. I must keep busy (some would say a workaholic) just to keep the nagging, intrusive desire at bay. I am constantly jealous of my family and friends and strangers who were content with their daily lives. I would question them all the time trying to figure out their secret and only frustrated myself more with their benign answers. I just can't figure out the point of life if this is it. It seems like we are missing something. I've always been a black and white person, I don't do well with the grey areas. I like absolutes. I like answers. I have been told by some people that if I had religious faith, it would be easier because I would just "know" but that reasoning has never sat well with me and only opens up 1000 more unanswered questions.

This quest led me to move locations 17 times since leaving home because the initial excitement of finding a new place in a new city and getting a new job and meeting new co-workers and friends would put my insatiable searching on the back burner for a while and give me some temporary peace. I was even up-front during job interviews and tell them I would only commit to 2 years. This garnered me lots of surprised, strange looks but also appreciation of my honesty. I also avoided serious commitment in relationships because I felt it was never fair to them. After dating for awhile, they would invariably start talking long term and I would close down. They wanted the white picket fence and 2.3 kids, and I wanted them to have it - with someone else. Someone who wanted it too and would give them what they needed. Don't get me wrong, I also dated some losers and certifiable nut jobs, who were not so deserving, but maybe that's why I dated them. There was no chance of a future with them and deep down, I knew it, so it took the pressure off.

I have worked in the veterinary field for 3 decades because animal welfare has been a crystal-clear passion of mine since a very young age. However, I have moved around within the field - large animal practice, small animal practice, exotics, shelters, horse farms, dairy farms - to keep it interesting. I also branched out in part time work in a construction site and bartending to spice it up a little. Temporary fixes.

The only thing that made a difference was having my son. Even though my entire world was turned upside down all around me and was full of negative, fearful, stressful BS, becoming his mother was the most rock solid, 1000% commitment I had ever made, and it felt RIGHT. I now understood that old adage "don't mess with Mama bear" on so many levels. There is nothing more primal, more all encompassing, more important and more amazing.

As age and experience kept adding up (and up and up), I started being more conscious of my choices and decisions. I still haven't found "it", but I do know now that "it" doesn't come from a job, a location, or another person. I have really enjoyed writing this book and reliving some old stories and my intention is that it will help some people and brighten their day. This writing experience has definitely been interesting and feels "right" but I'm still on the hunt for something. Throughout my life and all my experiences, I always assumed that "Murphy's Law" had a real hate on for me and really thrived on screwing me over. As each new hurdle came to me, I would grit my teeth, shake my head, curse him and soldier on. I came to expect that life would never be easy for me. In my circle of friends and family, common statements were, "Oh shit, Murphy got you again!" or "Man, only you Stacy!" or "Do you ever catch a break?!" or "Come on! Not again!". Of course, there are people who have it much worse, but not as many who seem to have seen the consistency of Murphy's sick sense of humor. I've always wondered why I've had so many bad/sad/crazy experiences in my life but I guess it was so I could write this! It would have been pretty boring otherwise.

While putting this book together, I've slowly been realizing that not everyone can be Mother Theresa, Brad Pitt, Michael Jordan or the Rolling Stones but that doesn't make any of us less important. Those selected few have an impact on millions but sometimes having an impact on just one person can be just as powerful.

I realize that my sense of humour, writing style and potty mouth aren't for everyone – and that's OK. But if I can open up and share some of my crazy life and that in turn can make someone smile or help them feel less alone then that's a hell of a great thing. We don't all have to become household names, but we do all need to contribute what we have. This is what I have.

If anyone out there figures out how to find "it" please let me know. While I'm waiting, I will keep plugging away and see what I find.

Author Biography

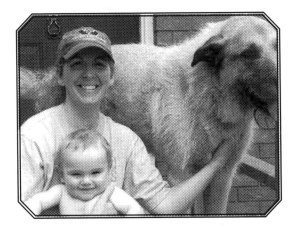

Stacy Cloran is a Mom, a Registered Veterinary Technician and a bed rest warrior and survivor. After serving an 87 day hospitalized bed rest sentence during her pregnancy, she found there was a definite lack of humorous support (especially when renting the hospital TV/phone/internet was $20/day....87x$20 - you do the math). During those 3 months she decided to help others stuck in similar situations by writing about her ordeal and recounting some of her unique life experiences to keep you entertained.